Practical Ways to Improve Patient Adherence

The *New York Times* has called adherence the world's "other drug problem." Physicians prescribe medications, but patients do not always use them. While it would be easy for physicians to blame patients for treatment failures, physicians can do more to motivate patients to use their medications as recommended.

Practical Ways to Improve Patient Adherence, Second Edition, is an excellent resource for physicians and allied health professionals whose patients exhibit poor adherence. Daniel J. Lewis, MD (Department of Dermatology, University of Pennsylvania Health System), and experienced adherence researcher Steven R. Feldman, MD, PhD (Departments of Dermatology and Social Sciences & Health Policy, Wake Forest University School of Medicine), examine the problem of poor adherence and offer concrete techniques to encourage patients to use their medications and improve treatment outcomes.

This book offers novel, potent ways to get patients to use their medications and improve treatment outcomes—tools healthcare providers can use day in and day out. A medical education is not complete without a thorough understanding of the hurdles that contribute to poor adherence and what health professionals can and should do about it.

20 years of patient adherence research presented in a simple, fun, and easy-to-read style . . . a once-in-a-lifetime treat!

Warren H. Chan, MD, MS, Dermatologist

Easy to digest and remarkably practical for physicians. . . . Recommend it to all my friends in medicine!

Diego R. Dasilva, MD, Dermatologist

Named the winner of the 2022 "Best Overall" Dermie Award by the *Dermasphere* podcast.

Published in association with the *Journal of Dermatological Treatment*.

SERIES IN DERMATOLOGICAL TREATMENT

About the Series

Published in association with the *Journal of Dermatological Treatment*, the *Series in Dermatological Treatment* keeps readers up to date with the latest clinical therapies to improve problems with the skin, hair, and nails. Each volume in the series is prepared separately and typically focuses on a topical theme. Volumes are published on an occasional basis, depending on the emergence of new developments.

Practical Ways to Improve Patient Adherence, Second Edition
Daniel J. Lewis and Steven R. Feldman

Atlas of Genital Dermoscopy
Giuseppe Micali and Francesco Lacarrubba

Hair Disorders: Diagnosis and Management
Alexander C. Katoulis, Dimitrios Ioannides, and Dimitris Rigopoulos

Techniques in the Evaluation and Management of Hair Disease
Rubina Alves and Juan Grimalt

Retinoids in Dermatology
Ayse Serap Karadag, Berna Aksoy, and Lawrence Charles Parish

Facial Skin Disorders
Ronald Marks

Dermatologic Reactions to Cancer Therapies
Gabriella Fabbrocini, Mario E. Lacouture, and Antonella Tosti

Acne Scars: Classification and Treatment, Second Edition
Antonella Tosti, Maria Pia De Padova, Gabriella Fabbrocini, and Kenneth Beer

Phototherapy Treatment Protocols, Third Edition
Steven R. Feldman and Michael D. Zanolli

Dermatoscopy in Clinical Practice: Beyond Pigmented Lesions, Second Edition
Giuseppe Micali and Francesco Lacarrubba

For more information about this series please visit: *www.crcpress.com/Series-in-Dermatological-Treatment/book-series/CRCSERDERTRE*

Practical Ways to Improve Patient Adherence

Second Edition

Daniel J. Lewis, MD
Department of Dermatology
University of Pennsylvania Health System

Steven R. Feldman, MD, PhD
Departments of Dermatology and Social
Sciences & Health Policy
Wake Forest University School of Medicine

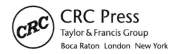

CRC Press
Taylor & Francis Group
Boca Raton London New York

CRC Press is an imprint of the
Taylor & Francis Group, an **informa** business

Designed cover image: Shutterstock

Second edition published 2024
by CRC Press
6000 Broken Sound Parkway NW, Suite 300, Boca Raton, FL 33487–2742

and by CRC Press
4 Park Square, Milton Park, Abingdon, Oxon, OX14 4RN

CRC Press is an imprint of Taylor & Francis Group, LLC

© 2024 Daniel J. Lewis, and Steven R. Feldman

Library of Congress Cataloging-in-Publication Data
Names: Lewis, Daniel J., author. | Feldman, Steven R., author.
Title: Practical ways to improve patient adherence / Daniel J. Lewis, Steven R. Feldman.
Other titles: Series in dermatological treatment.
Description: Second edition. | Boca Raton : CRC Press, 2023. | Series: Series in dermatological treatment |
   Includes bibliographical references and index.
Identifiers: LCCN 2023004580 (print) | LCCN 2023004581 (ebook) | ISBN 9781032435022 (hardback) |
   ISBN 9781032435015 (paperback) | ISBN 9781003367628 (ebook)
Subjects: MESH: Medication Adherence | Quality Improvement | Patients—psychology | Skin Diseases—
   drug therapy
Classification: LCC R726.5 (print) | LCC R726.5 (ebook) | NLM W 85 | DDC 610.1/9—dc23/eng/20230407
LC record available at https://lccn.loc.gov/2023004580
LC ebook record available at https://lccn.loc.gov/2023004581

ISBN: 978-1-032-43502-2 (hbk)
ISBN: 978-1-032-43501-5 (pbk)
ISBN: 978-1-003-36762-8 (ebk)

DOI: 10.1201/9781003367628

Typeset in Times
by Apex CoVantage, LLC

I dedicate this book to my parents, Iona and Leonard Lewis, particularly my mother, who has sacrificed countless hours over the last 25 years as I have continually worked to perfect my writing skills. She will always be the greatest English teacher in my life. I also dedicate the book to my amazing academic mentors—ranging from Dr. Madeleine Duvic and Dr. Steven R. Feldman in medical school to Dr. William Higgins and Dr. Christopher Miller during residency—for fostering my strong passion for academic dermatology, which I hope to continue building during my career.

Daniel J. Lewis, MD

I dedicate this book to my academic mentors, colleagues, research staff and fellows, and patients, all of whom have contributed the ideas and sweat that have made my understanding of adherence what it is today. I also dedicate the book to my parents, Ed and Fran Feldman, who supported my early learning and career development, and my wife Leora Henkin, and our sons, Jacob and Noah, who have taught me much about adherence and life over the years.

Steven R. Feldman, MD, PhD

Contents

Section 1 The Problem of Poor Adherence

Section 2 Foundation—Trust and Accountability

Section 3 Practicality—Simplicity and Education

Section 4   Psychology—Behavioral Techniques

Section 5   Special Considerations

Section 6   Illustrative Cases

Section 7   Final Thoughts

Authors

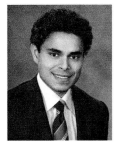

Daniel J. Lewis, MD is a Dermatology Chief Resident Physician in the Cutaneous Oncology track at the Perelman School of Medicine at the University of Pennsylvania. Dr. Lewis earned a BA in biology from the University of Pennsylvania, earned his MD at Baylor College of Medicine, and completed his internship at Memorial Sloan Kettering Cancer Center. He is a member of the Alpha Omega Alpha Honor Medical Society. He has authored over 75 peer-reviewed manuscripts as well as multiple textbook chapters. He was named Post-Doctoral Trainee of the Year in 2022 by ADEN and winner of the 2022 ASDS Young Investigators Writing Competition. He will be the 2023–2024 Micrographic Surgery and Dermatologic Oncology Fellow at the University of Pennsylvania.

Dr. Lewis also works as a professional sports journalist and has written over 90 articles for Yahoo! *Sports*, *Bleacher Report*, and *SB Nation* (www.DanielLewisSports.com). He is also Founder of Penn Fitness for Life, a community service organization based in Philadelphia that seeks to combat the growing obesity epidemic in the United States by empowering children to live healthy lives.

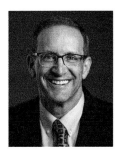

Steven R. Feldman, MD, PhD is Professor of Dermatology, Pathology, and Social Sciences & Health Policy, and Director of the Center for Dermatology Research at the Wake Forest University School of Medicine in Winston-Salem, North Carolina. He has authored over 1,200 peer-reviewed articles and has served as the principal investigator of industry, foundation, and federally funded studies.

Dr. Feldman has been ranked by ExpertScape as one of the top five worldwide experts in psoriasis, dermatology, and treatment adherence. He has served as a member of the medical board of the National Psoriasis Foundation, chaired that board's subcommittee on education, and served as Director of the Foundation's Chief Residents' Meeting on psoriasis treatment. He has also chaired the American Academy of Dermatology's Psoriasis Education Initiative Workgroup. He was the founder of www.DrScore.com and Chief Science Officer of Causa Research. He is Senior Advisor, Dermatology & Patient Adherence, for Sensal Health. He serves as the editor of or an editorial board member for multiple dermatology journals and is the author of *Compartments: How the Brightest, Best Trained, and Most Caring People Can Make Judgments That Are Completely and Utterly Wrong.* He is also the curator of www.PromisedLandMuseum.org, the Jewish Museum of the Palestinian Experience.

1

Introduction

Have you ever encountered a patient with a common skin disorder who stated, "Doctor, you are the sixth dermatologist I have seen for my condition?" Perhaps this patient had a particularly resistant skin condition, an unusual disease variant that did not respond to treatment the way the condition usually does, or perhaps the skills of the previous dermatologists the patient had visited were questionable. But think about it for a moment—what is the chance that a patient could see five other dermatologists, and not one of them made the correct diagnosis? That is rather unlikely. And what is the chance that a patient could see five other dermatologists, and not one of them prescribed the right treatment, even by chance? That is very unlikely too. There are so many caring, well-trained dermatologists, every one of whom would have made the right diagnosis and prescribed an appropriate treatment.

Still, it happens not infrequently that patients visit with that kind of story. What could be happening? Could patients with psoriasis somehow have inflammatory cells with mutated steroid receptors? Could patients be making antibodies against virtually every biologic therapy? Understanding how patients like these could fail treatment so many times is central to identifying the issues that contribute to treatment failure. Many patients who say, "Doctor, you are the sixth dermatologist I have seen for this" probably have one aspect in common that explains why their disease is so resistant to treatment. They probably are not using their medication as recommended.

The term *compliance* refers to how well patients use their medication. It is a term that was often taught in medical school, but it is now considered outdated and has largely been replaced with the term *adherence*. *Compliance* suggests that patients should bow to an authoritarian doctor figure, whereas the term *adherence* implies that patients actively engage in maintaining their health.

Poor adherence is ubiquitous in medicine, particularly in dermatology (Balkrishnan, 2005). The central thesis of this book is that we can and should improve our patients' treatment outcomes by getting them to use their medication better. Perhaps we can provide better patient care simply by encouraging patients to use the therapies we already have than we can by developing new ones. We may even be able to cure or clear patients of their disease with medications they have already tried—but did not use consistently or correctly—without resorting to riskier, more complicated, or costlier treatment regimens.

Patients are suffering from their medical conditions. We cannot assume that that suffering implies they will use treatment as recommended. This book is devoted to providing numerous practical approaches to alleviating suffering and helping patients better control their conditions through better use of their treatment.

Providing quality medical care involves three key aspects: making the right diagnosis, prescribing the appropriate treatment, and getting patients to use their medication. While poor adherence is very common, current medical school and residency training curricula largely ignore adherence issues. Medical training focuses on the first two aspects of good medical care—the diagnosis and treatment—even though the latter two—treatment and adherence—are more important in helping our patients get well. We learn about all sorts of pathologies and their respective treatments. Our pharmacology courses cover the absorption, distribution, and metabolism of drugs. But our training lacks a course that covers the principal factor that determines most of the variation in blood levels among patients. This variation is due, in large part, to variation in adherence—how well or how poorly patients follow the treatment plans we recommend.

In Dr. Ben Barankin's book *Dermographies: Autobiographies in Dermatology, Volume 2*, Dr. Stuart Maddin reported that his best piece of advice came from Dr. Marion Sulzberger, who "encouraged his residents to always be able to provide one further worthwhile treatment for the patient. He emphasized that having such depth was really the sign of a true consultant" (Barankin, 2006). Perhaps it would have been better advice to suggest that to be a great consultant, one must always possess one additional technique to get patients to use their medication.

This book is not intended to present a detailed theoretical analysis of patients' adherence behavior, nor is it intended to provide a comprehensive review of adherence research. The objective of this book is to give you quick, practical tips to help you improve your patients' adherence and their treatment outcomes.

Section 1

The Problem of Poor Adherence

DOI: 10.1201/9781003367628-2

2

How Poor Is Patient Adherence?

Patients' adherence to treatment encompasses multiple steps. After we give patients a prescription (or send it directly to their pharmacy so they do not lose it), they may or may not fill the prescription. If they do, they may or may not start the treatment. If they start the treatment, they may use it well or poorly, and they may discontinue the treatment before they are supposed to do so. Primary adherence refers to whether they start the treatment; secondary adherence comprises those behaviors after initiating treatment.

We view adherence through the perspective of our specialty: dermatology. Dermatology is an excellent model because many of the conditions we treat are chronic, and we also frequently prescribe topical treatment. Adherence to topical treatment is particularly difficult, making dermatologic treatment an excellent model for identifying poor adherence and developing new techniques to improve adherence.

Although research on adherence remains relatively limited in dermatology, other fields have studied it extensively while also assessing its impact on patient outcomes and identifying methods of improving patient adherence. Data on adherence to treatment for several non-dermatologic conditions—diabetes mellitus, sexually transmitted diseases, epilepsy, and asthma—provide a basis for understanding adherence in dermatology, which is likely worse than that seen in other fields of medicine.

2.1 Diabetes Mellitus

Like many dermatologic conditions, diabetes mellitus is a chronic disease that requires lifelong treatment. The pathogenesis of diabetes is well understood—it is a condition in which there is an absence of or resistance to insulin. Its diagnosis is also fairly straightforward as there are specific laboratory testing criteria for its diagnosis. There are also several excellent treatments for the disease. Those patients who lack insulin can receive recombinant insulin injections. For patients who are resistant to insulin, measures such as diet, exercise, and medications can reduce the degree of insulin resistance. The main issue in treating diabetes involves getting patients to make the lifestyle modifications that these treatments require.

Diabetes, if uncontrolled, can lead to serious consequences—blindness, cardiovascular disease, neurologic disease, kidney failure, and even limb amputation. Given these potentially horrible consequences, it would be logical to think that patients would adhere well to recommended treatment. However, the prevalence

DOI: 10.1201/9781003367628-3

of uncontrolled diabetes demonstrates that patients can have a very serious disease with life-threatening consequences yet still not use treatment as recommended.

It is not enough for us to have medications to treat diabetes; we must also encourage patients to use them. We must counsel them effectively so that they incorporate taking their medication and monitoring their blood glucose into their daily routines. In this sense, the most important advances in the treatment of diabetes have focused on minimizing the burden of treatment. Superior delivery systems—insulin pens and pumps as well as long-acting treatments such as insulin glargine—and less invasive techniques to monitor blood glucose levels are innovations that facilitate better patient management of diabetes. Dermatology patients might also benefit if these concepts were incorporated into the treatment of their skin disease. More broadly, all patients might benefit if these concepts were incorporated throughout medicine.

Another important lesson from the example of diabetes relates to disease assessment. Since diabetes involves elevated blood glucose levels, it would seem that measuring the blood glucose level in the doctor's office would be the number one way to assess the severity of disease. In reality, measuring blood glucose is a poor way to assess glucose control as it only provides information about glucose levels at that very moment. Patients with diabetes may have excellent glucose control during an office visit but not at other times—a very common phenomenon, one that we will return to and discuss in greater detail. Patients' behavior is substantially different preceding an office visit, affecting the severity of their illness when they are seen by the physician. In diabetes, measuring a hemoglobin A1C level, which provides a snapshot of the blood glucose level over a three-month period, allows the physician to assess glucose control between appointments. More such measures are needed to assess how well patients use their treatments over the long stretches of time between doctor office visits.

2.2 Sexually Transmitted Infections

A common myth is that when patients have a symptomatic disease—one that bothers them a lot—they will adhere to treatment well. The care of patients with sexually transmitted diseases teaches us otherwise. Consider gonorrhea. One might assume that a patient with gonorrhea—characterized by painful, purulent genital discharge—would be bothered by their disease. The condition might affect them psychologically and socially. Presumably, they would want to get rid of it as soon as possible and wouldn't want it to recur. More than just theoretically, patients with gonorrhea ought to be highly motivated to treat their disease given its stigma, its effects on their social behaviors, and the symptoms of a painful, purulent discharge. The treatment is easy! Gonorrhea can be treated effectively if patients take an oral antibiotic twice a day for just one week. Yet patients with gonorrhea often fail to take the recommended oral antibiotic for even a single week. For this reason, gonorrhea is treated by the administration of an intramuscular antibiotic. In dermatology, patients have symptomatic conditions that impair quality of life, but are they worse than "the clap?" The recommended treatment regimens in dermatology are typically far more complex and time consuming than taking an oral antibiotic twice a day for one week. We cannot assume that just because patients have a severely symptomatic illness, they will adhere to treatment.

Skin diseases cause patients to experience significant suffering. Patients can develop intractable pruritus that interferes with sleep. The appearance of lesions and the reactions of other people upon seeing the lesions can be devastating to patients. One might assume that because skin disease is so distressing, dermatology patients would adhere to treatment. However, if patients with a condition as psychologically distressing as gonorrhea do not take an oral antibiotic reliably for just one week, how much worse is adherence in patients with chronic skin diseases who are receiving topical therapies? In one study of patients with moderate-to-severe psoriasis, the worse the impact of their disease, the *worse* their adherence. Patient adherence should not be taken for granted. If anything, we should assume that non-adherence is the norm and work assiduously to promote adherence.

2.3 Epilepsy

Epilepsy is another condition that requires lifelong treatment. Many effective anticonvulsant drugs are available. Yet it is often difficult, particularly in children with epilepsy, to maintain control of the disease. Even patients who appear to use their medication well, as evidenced by adequate blood levels of their antiepileptic medication, may experience breakthrough seizures.

Poor adherence may represent the primary cause of breakthrough seizures. Why would a patient with an adequate blood level of the antiepileptic medication develop breakthrough seizures? A drug blood level only reflects the level at the time of the office visit, which only reflects adherence in the days prior to the office visit. Just as patients with diabetes may exhibit adequate glucose control during an office visit and inadequate control between visits, patients with epilepsy may take their medication regularly around the time of the office visit but not so regularly between visits. Drug blood levels provide information about adherence around the time the blood is drawn. Electronic adherence monitors would tell a different story—one of poor adherence between office visits.

2.4 Asthma

Adherence issues in treating children with asthma may be informative in treating children with atopic dermatitis and other conditions. Common strategies to optimize treatment outcomes have little to do with underlying genetic or immunologic issues. Fundamentally, both asthma and atopic dermatitis represent chronic diseases characterized by frequent flares. In both conditions, not only are there several treatments that may be prescribed at one time, but many of the treatments are also very complex. Even worse, the various treatments often require modification over time based on the ever-changing severity of the illness. The intricacies of treating these conditions are compounded by poor patient adherence.

Dr. Bruce Rubin, a pediatric pulmonologist, describes what asthma patients or their parents mean when they say, "My asthma medication is not working" (Rubin, 2004). With a few word substitutions, his descriptions would apply directly to children with atopic dermatitis. Although his classification scheme allows for the possibility of a physician making an incorrect diagnosis or prescribing an inappropriate treatment, he recognizes poor adherence as the cause of poor treatment outcomes. Dr. Rubin's classification scheme emphasizes that there may be several reasons why patients do not use their medication:

1. The patient does not want to take medication—the patient is not actually sick, the patient is seeking secondary gain, or the medication is too expensive.
2. The patient does not understand how or when to use medication.
3. The patient is concerned about medication side effects.
4. The patient cannot feel the medication working.
5. The patient has unrealistic expectations.
6. The patient incorrectly thinks that they are inhaling medication.
7. The patient does not have asthma.
8. The patient needs a stronger or additional medication.

Notice that most of Dr. Rubin's reasons for poor adherence are patient centered, a common way to frame the problem. However, perhaps a more practical way to frame the problem that will guide us to solutions is as a physician-centered one since we can control what we do. For example, the problem is not that our patients do not understand how or when to use medication; the problem is that we do not adequately communicate how and when to use the medication. We only have direct control over our own behavior, and so for us to solve the adherence problem, we have to change what we do.

3

Qualitative Measures of Adherence

3.1 Obtaining an Adherence History

Improving adherence in large part depends on being able to measure adherence. Unfortunately, there are very few accurate ways of assessing adherence in clinical practice. In general, the best approach might simply be to assume that our patients are not using their medication, especially when it is not working as well as we might have expected. We can attempt to obtain an adherence history, but patients will often report that they are taking their medication, even if they are not. Some patients might also tell their dentists they are flossing regularly even if they hardly floss at all. When comparing adherence data from objective electronic monitors (in the caps of medicine containers that record when patients open and close the container) to patients' treatment diaries, patients commonly overreport use of their medication. How can we assess this in our clinic patients?

3.1.1 Indirect Questioning

It may be compelling to ask patients if they are following the treatment plan. However, it may be best to avoid doing so in a way that might be perceived as confrontational. For example, directly asking, "Are you drinking alcohol?" might lead a patient to respond, "No," even if they are heavily drinking. Alternatively, we might ask, "How many cases of beer do you go through in a week?" In answering this question, the patient can proudly and honestly respond, "Doctor, I only drink a few beers on the weekend."

When asking whether patients have been taking their medication, consider instead asking how often they have not. We might ask, "How often do you miss doses? Every day or every other day?" This question frames missing occasional doses as acceptable, encouraging patients to be honest about their adherence. It also makes them feel proud of themselves when they can report missing a dose only once a week. Conversely, asking, "Have you been taking the medication?" leads patients to answer reflexively, "Yes, Doctor."

RECOMMENDED QUOTE

We should avoid asking, "Have you been taking the medication?" We are more likely to get an honest answer if we instead ask, "How often do you miss doses? Every day or every other day?"

DOI: 10.1201/9781003367628-4

This method of "indirect questioning" may lead to more accurate responses about adherence. The following are additional indirect, non-judgmental questions we can ask to evaluate our patients' adherence (Alinia and Feldman, 2014).

3.2 Adherence Assessment Questionnaire

1. Do you need a refill?
   - Yes
   - No
2. When you need a refill, what do you do?
   - Call the pharmacy
   - Go by the pharmacy
   - Use an online or other electronic refill system
   - Not applicable
3. If it is time for a refill and you still have extra medicine, what do you do?
   - Wait to fill the refill
   - Fill the refill anyway
   - Throw the old medicine away and get the refill
   - Not applicable
4. Does the pharmacy send you medication even when you don't need it?
   - Yes
   - No
   - Not applicable
5. Where do you keep extra (prescribed) medicine that has accumulated?
   - In the medicine cabinet
   - In the kitchen
   - In another room or location
   - I dispose of extra medicine
   - Not applicable
6. What do you do with extra medicine you accumulate? (circle all that apply):
   - Return it to the pharmacy
   - Donate it to charitable organizations
   - Share it with friends and relatives
   - Dispose of it
   - Not applicable
7. How do you dispose of unused medicine?
   - Down the sink
   - Down the toilet

- In the trash can
- Not applicable

8. Do you keep extra syringes of medication refrigerated?

- Yes
- No
- Not applicable

9. Is the cabinet where you keep extra medicine locked?

- Yes
- No
- Not applicable

The adherent patient would respond "not applicable" to these questions; most patients would give some other response.

There are some patients who are incredibly convincing in their protestations about their near-perfect adherence to treatment. When therapy is not working as well as expected, it may be best to trust patients yet still consider the possibility of poor use of the medication. The Cold War advice "Trust, but verify" may be appropriate.

3.2.1 Religiosity and Honesty

Behavioral economists who study honesty may have identified another approach we can use, recognizing individuals are generally more honest when they are placed in a religious frame of mind. Students cheated less on examinations after they were first asked to list as many of the Ten Commandments as they could. It did not matter how many of the commandments they listed, how many they got correct, or even if they were religious at all. Simply making them think about religion caused them to be more honest. Therefore, when we are caring for patients who we know are religious, priming them by first asking them about their church, mosque, or synagogue may yield more honest answers when we then ask them about their use of their medication. In theory, wearing a Ten Commandments tie and talking about it before asking about adherence might improve the accuracy of the information we receive.

3.2.2 Informal Auditing

For patients using self-administered biologics for psoriasis, we can deftly assess adherence by asking, "Are you keeping the extra injectors you have accumulated in the refrigerator like you are supposed to?" Adherent patients should answer, "Doctor, I am not really sure what you are talking about. I do not have any extra injectors." If patients instead respond affirmatively that they keep the extras refrigerated, we immediately know they are accumulating extras and must not be using the medication as prescribed. Similarly, when caring for patients on isotretinoin for acne, a good way to find out if adherence is poor may be to ask, "Do you have any extra isotretinoin pills you would be able to use to tide you over if there's a delay in seeing you between our monthly visits?"

RECOMMENDED QUOTE

For patients on biologics, we can assess adherence by asking, "Are you keeping the extra injectors you have accumulated in the refrigerator like you are supposed to?"

Dr. Keith Vaughan of University Place, Washington, suggests advising patients to bring their current medication regimen to their follow-up visit as part of an informal auditing process. This strategy is particularly helpful if we prescribed multiple medications at the initial visit or if we might expect adherence issues based on their demeanor or overall behavior. In reality, though, we should anticipate adherence issues at every visit.

3.3 Tube Weights and Pill Counts

In research studies assessing adherence to topical therapy, we can weigh the medication tubes. This method is not practical for everyday practice, but we can still assess patient adherence simply by looking at the medication. We can count pills or look at the tubes and clearly recognize that patients are not using the medication if the tube or bottle remains full, or the container indicates that the medication was never refilled. However, an empty tube or bottle does not necessarily mean patients used the medication; they may have simply dumped, squeezed, or poured it into their trash can at home.

Similarly, pill counts may be unreliable. If we want to assess adherence by using pill counts, we should not give patients 60 pills for twice-daily use and suggest they return in one month. If we do, an empty bottle might mean they either exhibited perfect adherence or threw out the pills. In one study using electronic monitors, a patient returned with an empty bottle and a self-recorded treatment diary indicating that she had taken the medication daily as prescribed (Krejci-Manwaring and Johnson, 2007). The electronic monitor showed that, in reality, she had only opened the bottle once, presumably to toss the pills into the trash can.

We can make pill counts more useful by prescribing more pills than patients would need. For example, we might prescribe 70 pills for twice-a-day use for one month or prescribe 60 pills and see the patient back in three weeks. If patients present an empty bottle at the return visit, then they likely threw the pills in the trash can. Meanwhile, if the bottle contains 10 pills, then they almost certainly must be using their medication very well.

3.4 Electronic Monitoring

Electronic monitors represent an excellent resource for assessing adherence. Aardex's Medication Event Monitoring System (MEMS) bottle caps (www.aardex group.com/solutions/mems-adherence-software/) record the date and time whenever the medication bottle is opened (**Figure 3.1**). Although these devices are very

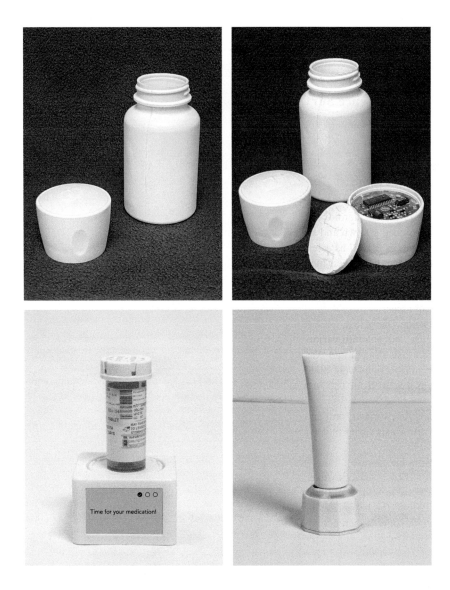

FIGURE 3.1 Electronically monitored bottle caps. The Medication Event Monitoring System (MEMS) bottle caps (top images) can provide detailed and objective information on how often patients use their medication. Newer medication devices from Sensal (bottom images) can record the time of administration and the change in container weight for both oral (dock) and topical (smart cap) dosage forms.

practical for clinical research studies, they are costly and not practical for everyday clinic use.

3.5 Adherence Survey Studies in Dermatology

Before the development of electronic monitors, adherence in dermatology had been measured primarily via surveys. One survey asked patients with psoriasis how well they had been using their medication. The survey was anonymous, so patients should have felt comfortable providing an honest report. Nearly 40% admitted to not using their medication as directed (Richards and Fortune, 1999); we suspect most of the other 60% were not telling the truth. A similar survey assessing the use of topical steroids for psoriasis also found that 40% of subjects reported poor adherence (Brown and Rehmus, 2006). Frustrations related to efficacy and inconvenience as well as a fear of side effects were among the most common reasons they did not use their medication. Other factors included cost, unclear instructions, overly complicated directions, and the unpleasant feeling of the medication.

Since Denmark maintains a national pharmacy database, researchers in Denmark can assess how long patients take to fill their prescriptions, if they fill them at all. In one Danish study, dermatologists had written prescriptions for medications to treat patients with various skin diseases—acne, atopic dermatitis, infections, and psoriasis (Storm and Andersen, 2008). About 90% of prescriptions for acne and skin infections were filled within one month; many people think that sounds good, but it is far from a six-sigma level of quality—if only 90% of Toyota cars worked, we would be far from satisfied. For atopic dermatitis, only two-thirds were filled, and for psoriasis, only half the prescriptions were filled!

Psoriasis varies in its severity and its effects on patients' lives. We might assume that patients with severe psoriasis would try the hardest to reduce their suffering from the disease. Nevertheless, in one study, patients with severe disease—as measured by disease involvement or its impact on quality of life—were *less likely to adhere to treatment* than those with mild disease (Zaghloul and Goodfield, 2004). Perhaps the brain does not want to think about severe disease or the treatment of it. In short, adherence can be highly unpredictable, and we should avoid making conjectures about adherence without testing our predictions.

4

Clinical Studies on Adherence

Assessing patient adherence—whether by pill counts or patient-reported treatment diaries—poses significant limitations. Patients often report having used far more medication than they have actually used. Pill counts and tube weights are similarly unreliable because patients may have dumped the medication into their trash cans at home. On the other hand, electronic monitoring devices—used in studies to assess adherence in patients with HIV infection, diabetes, epilepsy, and asthma—offer a more accurate, objective method of assessing adherence. Those studies show that adherence is less than what patients self-report. Adherence studies done in dermatology show similar findings.

4.1 Psoriasis

Psoriasis is a chronic disease that can frustrate both us and our patients. Finding a sufficiently effective therapy can be difficult, and our treatments seem to lose efficacy over time. Some of the earliest adherence research in dermatology involved patients with psoriasis. One early study assessed patients' use of 6% salicylic acid gel, which was administered in an attempt to potentiate the effects of 0.1% Protopic (tacrolimus) ointment (Carroll, 2005). Topical tacrolimus is effective in treating psoriasis affecting the face or intertriginous areas, and perhaps topical tacrolimus might also be effective in treating plaque psoriasis in other areas if combination use with salicylic acid were to promote greater penetration.

In the study, subjects were given tacrolimus ointment to apply to their lesions on both sides of the body for eight weeks. They were also instructed to apply salicylic acid gel twice a day to their plaques but to use it only on one side of the body, allowing for left-right comparisons. The salicylic acid was provided in containers equipped with electronic monitors. Subjects were informed that they were being monitored and were asked to maintain a medication diary and bring their medication bottles to clinic for weighing. However, they were not told about the electronic monitors in the medication bottle caps.

The use of electronic monitors opened a window into the previously unseen aspects of patient adherence in the treatment of psoriasis. Some patients used the salicylic acid nearly as recommended. One particularly obsessive-compulsive patient documented using it exactly as the electronic monitor indicated (Balkrishnan and Carroll, 2003). Other patients did not use it nearly as well. Two subjects reported using it as directed but used it rarely according to the monitors. One subject presented to the clinic complaining of signs of salicylism—tinnitus, difficulty with

DOI: 10.1201/9781003367628-5

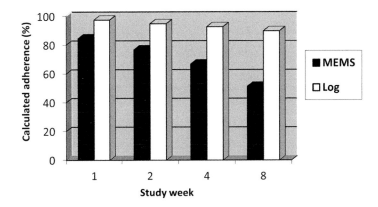

FIGURE 4.1 **Weekly use of 6% salicylic acid gel in combination with 0.1% tacrolimus ointment in patients with psoriasis.** The electronically monitored bottle caps showed that patients used their medication less often than they indicated in their diaries. Interestingly, use of the medication decreased by 20% every five weeks; the decreasing use of medication over time likely leads to loss of efficacy, a phenomenon often interpreted clinically as "tachyphylaxis." Abbreviation: MEMS, Medication Event Monitoring System.

balance—which were worrisome until the researchers noted the subject had only opened the container once, which would not have been enough applications to cause salicylism. Based on these findings, we can only wonder how much more effective drugs might be in clinical trials if clinical trial subjects used them more reliably.

According to the treatment diaries, subjects applied more than 90% of the prescribed doses of salicylic acid over the eight-week study period (**Figure 4.2**). However, according to the electronic monitors, while they used it well on the first day, their use declined dramatically, by about 40%, over the next few days (Carroll and Feldman, 2004). Adherence then continued to decrease slowly over time, aside from brief increases occurring at two-week intervals. What accounted for these regular increases? The study visits. Just as individuals tend to floss their teeth more often just before seeing the dentist, patients use their medications in the days before they come to see us for office visits. The adherence literature terms this "white coat compliance," but we prefer to call it "the dental floss phenomenon."

In the salicylic acid study, adherence decreased by 20% every five weeks. Although the study only lasted eight weeks and extrapolating beyond the range of the data is a dubious endeavor, we might infer that if the adherence were to continue to decrease by 20% every five weeks, adherence would reach zero after 25 weeks, or after about six months. (It is generally a mistake to extrapolate beyond the range of the data, but we do so here for illustrative purposes.) In dermatology, we have a name for when adherence to topical therapy approaches zero. We call it "tachyphylaxis." When patients with psoriasis or atopic dermatitis were given a topical steroid, it was common for it to work well at first but to gradually lose efficacy over time. The loss of effectiveness was called tachyphylaxis. The dogma was that tachyphylaxis meant "the more you use the steroid, the less it works," potentially due to a downregulation of steroid receptors. But after seeing what happens with adherence over time,

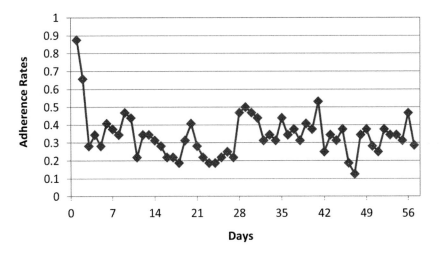

FIGURE 4.2   Daily use of 0.1% triamcinolone ointment in children with atopic dermatitis.
Although patients used the triamcinolone ointment on the first day of the study, adherence
plummeted over the next two days and then continued to decrease. The rate at which adherence
declines likely correlates with the rate at which "tachyphylaxis" develops.

tachyphylaxis clearly means "the *less* you use the steroid, the less it works." Before
this study, dermatologists were unaware of how patients actually used their medication, and so we simply believed patients when they claimed, "Doctor, I have been
using the medication religiously. It just does not work anymore."

One way we could prove that tachyphylaxis is due to poor adherence would be to
conduct a study in which we gave triamcinolone to patients with localized plaque
psoriasis. We could give them the medication in blue bottles equipped with electronic monitors. Then, when the medication inevitably stopped working, we could
administer the same medication in red bottles and demonstrate that it started working again. But we already do something similar in our practices. When patients
develop "tachyphylaxis," we often switch to another steroid of the same class.
If tachyphylaxis were due to the downregulation of steroid receptors, when one
mid-potency steroid stopped working, the others should not work either (Ali and
Brodell, 2007).

The idea that tachyphylaxis is due to poor adherence was tested in a small study
that enrolled patients who had failed topical steroids for their psoriasis (Okwundu
and Cardwell, 2021); a similar study was done in patients with atopic dermatitis
(Okwundu and Cardwell, 2018). The patients were given an easy-to-use topical
steroid under conditions designed to get them to use the product. (There were many
return visits designed to drive them to use the medication.) These patients who
had previously failed topical steroids all improved. While the studies were small,
the findings suggest that most "tachyphylaxis" with topical steroids is due to poor
adherence to the treatment.

Consistent with the idea that tachyphylaxis is due to poor adherence, another
small study examined adherence to long-term use of a potent topical steroid for

psoriasis (Alinia and Moradi Tuchayi, 2017). Patients were given topical fluocinonide 0.05% to apply twice daily and were followed for a year. Use of the medication, assessed with electronic monitors, decreased rapidly over the first month of the study. Over the last month of treatment, no medication was used on half the days of the month. Drug holidays of seven days or more without using the treatment were common, occurring in about one-third of subjects in the first month and in 40% in the twelfth month of the study. Patients took the prescribed dose on only about 20% of study days. Long-term adherence to topical treatment can be abysmal.

4.2 Atopic Dermatitis

Atopic dermatitis is another condition that is often complicated by poor patient adherence. For example, consider a child with extensive lichenified lesions affecting the entire body that are refractory to all sorts of outpatient therapies. If we were to admit this child to the hospital and treat the child with topical 0.1% triamcinolone ointment—perhaps along with anti-staphylococcal antibiotics, if indicated—the lesions would clear almost completely in just a few days. Hospitalization would lead to rapid improvement, not because it removes the patient from the dust mites at home or somehow "takes patients away from the stress of the home environment," but rather because hospitalization helps ensure that the triamcinolone is applied.

A "real-life" trial assessed adherence to topical triamcinolone in children with atopic dermatitis (Krejci-Manwaring and Tusa, 2007). Patients and their parents were given 0.1% triamcinolone ointment and were instructed to use it twice a day. The medication was provided in bottles equipped with electronic monitors. Patients were told to return in one month. They were not told about the electronic monitors. For the investigators to learn what adherence was like in real life, the research subjects were not even told they were part of a study!

In the adherence study on psoriasis described here, patients did not use their topical medications very well. We have to wonder how much worse adherence is in real-life clinical practice than it was in the research study. The psoriasis study included a number of factors—patients knowing that they were being monitored, filling out treatment diaries, coming in for return visits every two weeks, receiving written instructions, and being compensated for their participation—that should have motivated the subjects to use their medication better than they would in everyday practice. Accordingly, to understand what patient adherence is like in real-life patients, unlike in the psoriasis study, patients in this real-life atopic dermatitis study were not told that they were part of a trial. There was no consent form. If the patients had known that they were part of a study, it might have affected their behavior, a principle known as the Hawthorne effect (Davis and Feldman, 2013).

In the study, use of triamcinolone was excellent on the first day (**Figure 4.2**). However, over the next three days, adherence dropped by 60–70%. It continued to decrease over time, but then it suddenly increased at one month—at the time of the return office visit.

Poor adherence in children with atopic dermatitis should not be surprising. In treating pediatric patients, there are now multiple parties who can contribute to poor adherence: the child and caregivers. If you have ever tried putting sunscreen or a topical medication on your child, you likely understand why adherence is often so poor in pediatric patients.

An open-label study was performed in children with atopic dermatitis to evaluate whether measures aimed at improving adherence would yield better treatment outcomes (Yentzer and Camacho, 2010). The study participants were given desonide gel, a low-potency, easy-to-apply steroid. They also received written instructions to help them understand the medication. Subjects were told that they were being given a "cortisone-type" medication, without using the word "steroid," which conjures fear in many parents. In addition to a return visit in one week, patients were contacted by phone three days after they began treatment to inquire about their use of the medication.

The interventions worked well. Patients reported a high degree of satisfaction with the aqueous gel vehicle. Moreover, whereas in the previous study, use of the triamcinolone ointment decreased by 60–70% within three days, use of the desonide gel in this study decreased by only 30% in the first week and was roughly 50% at the end of four weeks. Nearly all subjects had clinically meaningful improvement; mean Eczema Area and Severity Index (EASI) scores improved from baseline by approximately 60%.

One pediatric dermatology expert reported that for patients with treatment-resistant atopic dermatitis, he is not afraid to use ultrapotent topical steroids, add penetration enhancers, recommend wet wraps, or switch to potent systemic agents such as methotrexate or cyclosporine. How effective are these approaches when the mother is afraid to use low-to-medium-potency topical steroids? Can we expect her to apply an ultrapotent steroid if she is afraid of using a weaker one? Will she apply two medications or use wet wraps after she was reluctant or unable to use even one medication regularly? For disease that is "resistant" to treatment, we do not need to resort to higher potency steroids or more complicated treatment regimens. Simply getting patients to use their medication better, even a modestly potent topical steroid, can be very effective.

Is it really possible that adherence is so poor among children with atopic dermatitis when the condition causes so much suffering? Don't parents love their children enough to apply the medication? We know parents love their children, but that doesn't mean adherence is good. Children with acute leukemia are treated with induction chemotherapy to induce remission and are then prescribed oral 6-mercaptopurine (6-MP) to maintain remission. Certainly, parents don't want the leukemia to return. But poor adherence to 6-MP is common. In a survey, poor adherence was *self-reported* in 25% of patients (Kahn and Stevenson, 2022). A study using electronic monitors found that 84% of patients overreported their use of 6-MP at least some of the time (Landier and Chen, 2017). Another study using electronic monitors found that while many patients had good adherence, adherence dropped over time in others, and some just had very poor adherence altogether (Rohan and Drotar, 2015).

4.3 Hand Dermatitis

Applying a topical agent is generally more difficult than taking a pill. One study examined the use of tacrolimus ointment as maintenance therapy for hand dermatitis in patients who had received a three-week course of oral prednisone (Krejci-Manwaring and McCarty, 2006). Both the bottles containing the prednisone pills and the containers filled with tacrolimus ointment were equipped with electronic monitors. Patients were instructed to take the oral prednisone once daily for three weeks and apply the tacrolimus ointment twice daily for 12 weeks.

Use of oral prednisone was generally good; overall, patients missed only a few doses. Use of tacrolimus ointment, though, was worse and declined over the 12 weeks of treatment. Of note, patients appeared to use the topical treatment more frequently on the day of the visit in addition to a few days before and after the visit (**Figure 4.3**).

Assessments of the average adherence of the entire study group do not reveal the variation in adherence among subjects; adherence in individual patients varied tremendously. One subject opened the prednisone bottle only a single time, presumably to toss the pills into the trash can, as she returned with an empty bottle (Krejci-Manwaring and Johnson, 2007). Another patient, who had developed hand dermatitis due to obsessive hand washing, was also obsessive in using her tacrolimus ointment, applying it 8 to 14 times per day. In short, it is very difficult to

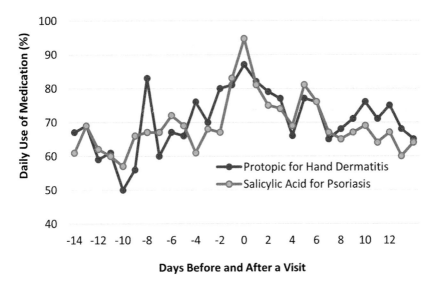

Days Before and After a Visit

FIGURE 4.3 **Medication use varies in relation to follow-up visits.** Patients' use of salicylic acid 6% gel for psoriasis and tacrolimus ointment for hand dermatitis was seemingly erratic. The percentage of patients who used their medication on a given day was plotted in relation to the day of the most recent or upcoming follow-up visit. Patients appeared to use their medication on the day of the visit in addition to a few days before and after the visit. They were far less likely to use their medication when there was no recent or upcoming follow-up visit.

predict how individual patients will use their medication; the potential range in behavior, from underuse to overuse, is enormous.

4.4 Acne

Although teenagers may be very bothered by their acne, they are not entirely adherent to treatment—not even close! Teenagers are particularly poor at seeking delayed gratification and may quickly give up on medications that do not produce rapid improvement. It's a vicious cycle as poor adherence contributes to poor outcomes that then contribute to poor adherence.

In one study (Yentzer and Alikhan, 2009), teenagers aged 13 to 18 were given benzoyl peroxide 5% gel to apply nightly for mild-to-moderate acne vulgaris for six weeks. Adherence averaged from 14% to 79%. Initially, about 8 in 10 subjects applied the medication on any given day; by the end of six weeks, only about 3 in 10 were applying the medication. Interestingly, only 11 of 19 subjects completed the study. If those who dropped out tended to be less adherent than the others, the data from this study probably overestimate the adherence of typical teenagers.

In another study, teenagers with acne were given Differin (adapalene) 0.1% gel in tubes equipped with electronic monitors (Yentzer and Gosnell, 2011). The study objective was to assess their adherence and evaluate interventions to improve their adherence. The study involved 60 patients, and all were instructed to apply the adapalene once daily for twelve weeks. One group—the standard-of-care group—was re-evaluated at six weeks and twelve weeks. Another group—the frequent-visit group—returned at one week, two weeks, four weeks, six weeks, eight weeks, and twelve weeks. This schedule was designed to mirror follow-up intervals in a standard clinical trial, hypothesizing that additional visits would promote better adherence. A third group—the electronic-reminder group—received a daily phone call to remind them to use their medication. The fourth group—the parental-reminder group—consisted of patients whose parents were called daily and were asked to remind the teen daily to use their medication.

In the standard-of-care group, adherence began at about 70% before decreasing to 40% over the course of the study (**Figure 4.4**). As expected, the frequent-visit group displayed the highest adherence, starting at about 80% before dropping to around 50% at the end of the study. The phone call reminders to the teenagers seemed to accomplish little; patients receiving these reminders exhibited adherence similar to that of the standard-of-care group. Interestingly, the parental reminder group showed the *worst* adherence of all four groups. Thus, in some patients, parental reminders may reduce teens' use of their medication.

4.5 Actinic Keratosis

Adherence is abysmal in children with atopic dermatitis, teenagers with acne, and young adults with psoriasis. How is adherence in older patients? In one study, patients with actinic keratoses were given fluorouracil 0.5% cream and were

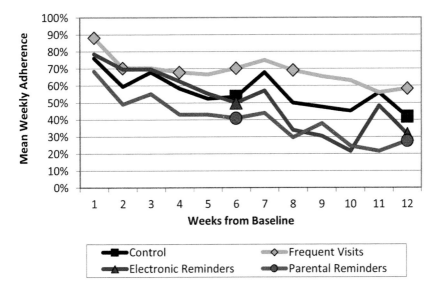

FIGURE 4.4   Weekly use of adapalene gel associated with various interventions in teenagers with acne. Patients were treated with adapalene gel daily for 12 weeks and divided into four groups based on the intervention they received to promote adherence. Frequent visits produced the highest level of adherence. Daily electronic reminders had little effect on adherence compared to the standard of care. Parental reminders yielded the worst adherence.

instructed to apply it daily for four weeks (Yentzer and Hick, 2009). They were also asked to complete a daily treatment diary and bring the medication to clinic for weighing. They were informed that they would be monitored but not that there were electronic monitors in the medication container caps. In contrast to the previous studies assessing adherence in psoriasis, atopic dermatitis, hand dermatitis, and acne, and despite the irritation that occurs with topical fluorouracil, adherence in this study was excellent. Roughly 90% of subjects were adherent, taking at least 80% of the recommended doses. In fact, on many occasions, when subjects missed a dose on one day, they used the medication twice the next day to make up for the missed dose.

The 5-fluorouracil cream is very irritating; one might have predicted that adherence would be terrible because of the potential for irritation. On the contrary, excellent adherence was observed. Several factors might explain the high level of adherence observed in this study. First, the duration of treatment was shorter than in some of the other studies, thus making adherence over the entire study period more feasible. Second, while we might think that patients would not use agents that cause irritation, the irritation might actually act as a constant reminder to use the medication, resulting in better adherence. The irritation may also make patients think the medication is working, encouraging them to continue using it. It is also possible that the nature of the disease drove adherence, as actinic keratoses are considered pre-cancerous lesions, and patients may be motivated by a fear of cancer. However, this possibility is not particularly likely, as motivation to get well does not seem to be a very good driver of adherence. Most importantly, though, perhaps older patients are simply more adherent than their younger counterparts. Older patients may be used to taking medications and may already have systems in place that remind them to do so.

5

Why Is Adherence So Poor? It Is Our Fault

Adherence researchers continue to wrestle with the question "Why is patient adherence so poor?" A number of patient and social support factors may contribute to poor adherence. Understanding potential barriers to adherence can help guide us in implementing strategies to help our patients use their medication. It may be that we need to look closer to home for answers.

5.1 Blame Ourselves, Not Our Patients

Our healthcare system in the U.S. is holding us increasingly responsible for our patients' outcomes. On the one hand, working to give our patients the best possible outcomes is what we want and expect from ourselves. On the other hand, we may wonder why we are held responsible when our patients are simply not using their medication.

It is perfectly reasonable for us to be held accountable for our patients' outcomes. Not only must we make the right diagnosis and prescribe the right treatment, but we must also encourage patients to use their medication. Poor adherence is primarily a *physician* problem, not a patient problem. While many physicians might disagree with this construct, holding ourselves responsible for poor adherence actually does us a service as the only way to change patient behavior is to change our own actions.

Much of the research on adherence has focused on how patient-related issues contribute to poor adherence. However, this perspective does not adequately describe our role in ensuring adherence. Attributing poor adherence to patients' lack of understanding, for example, undersells our responsibility to convey critical information in an effective manner. We can redefine several common patient barriers to adherence as physician or health system hurdles (**Table 5.1**) (Devine and Edwards, 2018).

While it is easy for us to write prescriptions, it is much harder for our patients to use the medications we prescribe. We may need to help them overcome multiple obstacles before they can successfully use their medication. In dermatology, we often prescribe topical agents, which require a higher level of dedication and precision, so it is far more difficult for us to get our patients to adhere to treatment than it is for physicians in other fields. Internalizing the skills to get patients to use a topical treatment would make us black belt experts at getting patients to use easier treatments like pills.

DOI: 10.1201/9781003367628-6

TABLE 5.1

Common Barriers to Patient Adherence Redefined as Physician or Health System Hurdles

Patient Barriers to Adherence	Physician or Health System Hurdles
Health literacy Education level Lack of knowledge of medication Concern about side effects	Inadequate transmission of information about condition or medication
Beliefs about medication Stigma or need for secrecy Cultural beliefs	Inadequate attention to aligning treatment with patient's beliefs and culture
View of symptoms ("Felt good, so did not take medication")	Inadequate education about need for treatment of asymptomatic disease
Medication abuse	Inadequate effort in addressing patient's substance abuse
Forgetting to take medication	Inadequate effort in helping patient set up reminder systems
Depression leading to poor motivation to take medication	Inadequate effort in identifying or addressing patient's depression
Cost and lack of insurance coverage	Prescribing unaffordable medications
Lack of caregiver	Inadequate attention to patient's support system
Lack of access to healthcare and resources	Inadequate provision of service at patient's location
Busy, competing priorities Changes to routine	Inadequate attention to patient's schedule when prescribing medication
Pill burden Complicated treatment regimen	Prescribing overly complex treatment regimens involving too many medications and a too-frequent dosing schedule

The Vietnamese Buddhist monk Thich Nhat Hanh shared valuable wisdom for life that is particularly apropos to our taking responsibility for patients' adherence to treatment:

> When you plant lettuce, if it does not grow well, you don't blame the lettuce. You look for reasons it is not doing well. It may need fertilizer, or more water, or less sun. You never blame the lettuce. Yet if we have problems with our friends or family, we blame the other person. But if we know how to take care of them, they will grow well, like the lettuce. Blaming has no positive effect at all, nor does trying to persuade using reason and argument. That is my experience. No blame, no reasoning, no argument, just understanding. If you understand, and you show that you understand, you can love, and the situation will change.

When the lettuce isn't growing well, you don't blame the patient. Hopefully nothing in this book has suggested that we should be blaming patients for poor adherence and resulting poor treatment outcomes. We need to do the things that will encourage better treatment adherence.

There are, perhaps rarely, some factors affecting adherence that remain out of our control. For instance, patients seeking disability may actively work to ensure that their condition does not improve. Nevertheless, there are many factors that we can control. As described in Chapter 9: Fostering Patient Accountability, the standard approach for getting patients to take medications is a model for failure. We can do better. The ensuing chapters describe practical ways for us to improve patient adherence.

6

A Pyramid Model for Improving Adherence

There are many reasons patients do not use their medication. Some adherence researchers argue that we must target our approach for improving adherence in an individual patient to the specific reason why they are non-adherent. While this method may work, a more general approach may be more effective. We can apply some general principles to encourage all patients to use their medication, regardless of their reasons for not using it.

The three levels for improving patient adherence are illustrated in **Figure 6.1**: (1) building a strong foundation centered on trust and accountability, (2) addressing practical issues to make treatment as easy as possible for our patients, and (3) utilizing specific behavioral techniques to give our patients an additional nudge to use their medication.

The first step in improving adherence entails building a foundation that fosters trust. Patients are cynical about insurance companies and the pharmaceutical industry; therefore, they must trust us before they will trust the medication we prescribe. Our patients will trust us only if they realize we care about them. We care about our patients, but the fact that we care about them has no impact on their behavior. None! Their behavior is determined solely by their *perception* of whether or not we care about them. Promoting trust and a sense that we care about them involves how we act and the context in which they see us act.

Once we establish a strong social bond with our patients, they will not want to let us down. Instead of fearing the medication, they may fear the embarrassment of not meeting the expectations of a physician who cares about them. Holding them accountable for the use of their medication—for example, with an office visit to see how well the treatment is working—is another component of the foundation on which adherence is built.

The second level involves making the treatment process as easy as possible for our patients. For one, we should always attempt to prescribe low-cost and fast-acting medications; combination drugs may be useful to simplify the treatment regimen for certain diseases. We can shorten the initial treatment interval to make the apparent burden of treatment appear lighter. Providing written instructions and suggesting patients use medication reminders are other simple measures that will empower patients to use their medication better.

The final level involves utilizing specific psychological techniques that encourage patients to follow their medication regimen. For example, recognizing that many patients exhibit an unreasonable fear of rare side effects, we can frame the risks of therapies in ways that put those risks into a more accurate perspective. In

DOI: 10.1201/9781003367628-7

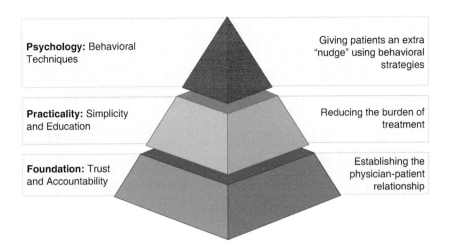

FIGURE 6.1 A pyramid model for improving adherence. The first step entails building a foundation centered on trust and accountability. The second step involves addressing practical issues to make the treatment process as easy as possible for patients. The final step involves employing practical psychological techniques to give patients an extra "nudge" to use their medication.

addition, a technique known as "anchoring" can make our patients less concerned about the burden of treatment. We can also use side effects to our advantage, proactively advising patients that a potential side effect is "a sign that the drug is working." By using these behavioral strategies, we can give patients a strong "nudge" to use their medication.

Section 2

Foundation—Trust and Accountability

DOI: 10.1201/9781003367628-8

7

Establishing the Physician–Patient Relationship

7.1 We Are Caring, But We Have to Show It

Medicine, at its heart, is a "people" business. We are not laboratory technicians following standardized protocols involving fixed quantities of highly purified reagents. It may seem that making accurate diagnoses and prescribing the appropriate treatment would be enough to help patients get well, but such is not the case.

While these duties are very important, we need to do more to be effective caregivers. We must also convey a sense of caring and trust. This aspect comes naturally to some doctors, whereas others do it with showmanship. There is nothing wrong with either approach. The key is to recognize the need for a strong doctor-patient relationship and work toward building one. If patients feel that we do not care and that they cannot trust us, they are not going to use the medications we prescribe, and they are not going to get well.

Some doctors may feel that their relationships with patients are their *raison d'être* for being doctors. However, for the rest of us, establishing a strong physician–patient relationship has a practical purpose. If we cultivate one, patients are more likely to use their medication; if we do not, they are less likely to do so. "Touchy-feely" doctors establish close, interpersonal relationships with patients automatically. For practical purposes, though, we do not have to be touchy-feely doctors for patients to view us as their allies. Those of us who got into medicine because we do well on standardized tests, not because of our social skills, just need to exhibit some of the behaviors that come naturally to the physician-humanist.

Vic Marks provides some excellent techniques in his article "Service Excellence in Dermatology" (**Table 7.1**) (Marks and Hutchison, 2004).

As Marks outlines, for patients who say they have taken several medications but still have active disease, we can empathize: "I bet the previous treatments have been very frustrating, right?" These words are very powerful. The patient will think we have read their mind, but in fact, patients are almost always frustrated by the previous treatment; if they had a treatment they liked that worked very well, they would not be sitting on our examination table with active disease.

DOI: 10.1201/9781003367628-9

TABLE 7.1

Service Excellence Skills: Showing We Care

First impressions count	Look patients in the eye when you meet them. Introduce yourself in an appropriate manner. Even before they meet you, make sure your front office communicates the right message.
Let patients tell you their stories	Do not interrupt if you can help it. Do not appear rushed.
Show you are listening	Look intently while patients speak. Ask questions to show your understanding. Restate what they say.
Touch their skin	Touching helps communicate a thorough examination was done. Using a lighted magnifying device such as a dermatoscope helps in this regard.
Explain the condition and the reason for treatment	Use understandable terminology.
Show empathy	Say something such as, "Your previous treatments have probably been frustrating."
Address psychosocial issues	Recommend support groups.
Solicit input and questions	Ask, "Do you have any other questions?" before ending the visit.
Make yourself accessible	Give your contact information to patients. Make sure there are appropriate policies in place in case patients have questions or concerns after the visit.

RECOMMENDED QUOTE

To show empathy for our patients, we can ask, "I bet the previous treatments have been very frustrating, right?"

7.1.1 Entering the Examination Room

Establishing trust begins before we start to examine the patient. Rushing to the exam room may help keep patients from waiting. But once arriving at that door, opening the door very slowly will help avoid giving patients the impression that we are rushed.

7.1.2 Hand Washing

Before shaking hands with patients (or bumping fists in the post-pandemic world), applying hand sanitizer is important. The spread of methicillin-resistant *Staphylococcus aureus* (MRSA) is a growing problem. We are told to wash our hands to help prevent the spread of the bacteria. Patients expect us to do it. If we wash our hands in the hallway and the patients do not see us do it, they might think we are infectious menaces.

More than just cleaning our hands, making patients remember that we did it is also important. We can do this by telling the patient, "Before I examine you, I have to apply this hand sanitizer. It's to protect you from doctor office germs like MRSA, flesh-eating bacteria, Ebola, Zika, evil humors, whatever that last patient had, and *monkeypox*." If we don't make the hand sanitizer use memorable, patients may have doubts about us when they hear stories of doctors who don't clean their hands. When it comes to changing patients' adherence behaviors, patients' perceptions are more important than reality.

Another dermatologist told us that after washing and drying his hands, he carries the used paper towels into the exam room and disposes of them in there, letting the patient see that he had just finished washing his hands. What a wonderful, practical way of making sure our patients witness a quality effort we make that might otherwise go unseen and unappreciated. We still like to use hand sanitizer in front of the patient. Describing the scary infections hopefully paints an unforgettable image in patients' minds that makes our use of hand sanitizer an unforgettable reminder of how we care for our patients. The unforgettable picture is an example of the concept of salience, which is discussed further in Chapter 15: Giving Salient Descriptions.

7.1.3 Facial Expressions and Body Language

Patients are silent observers of our facial and body language. They might recall a single discouraging statement or inappropriate facial expression that we made. These actions might negatively influence their opinion of us, even though our fund of knowledge or bedside manner might be otherwise stellar. Thus, communication skills are often more important than the diagnosis itself.

Speech characteristics such as rate, volume, pitch, and pauses also affect patients' perceptions of us. Non-verbal cues influence patients more often than verbal information. A blank expression is unwelcoming as it communicates disinterest and a lack of empathy. Nodding our heads, making eye contact, leaning forward, and smiling are all positive gestures that show attentiveness and are often well received. Similarly, praising patients for taking the initiative to come to the clinic also helps build rapport, especially when we consider that they often adjust their schedules to leave work or school to see us during normal clinic hours.

7.1.4 Physical Examination

One measure to ensure that patients trust us is to demonstrate that a thorough examination was performed. Conducting a complete skin examination in patients willing to have one done may be prudent. It may help to provide a written brochure on skin examination to inform patients why we are asking to perform the full examination. Touching the areas being examined helps us communicate to patients that we performed a thorough exam. When examining the back, the patient cannot tell what was or was not examined, so it may help to palpate the back as we look at it so the patient knows what parts were evaluated. When a patient points to a pigmented lesion and says, "This one is different from all my other spots. It has changed, and I am worried about it," we will almost undoubtedly need to perform a biopsy; even if it looks like a seborrheic keratosis, it might be an atypical melanoma. But before we perform the biopsy, we should nevertheless examine the lesion carefully using a lighted magnifying glass, such as a dermatoscope. Using such a device will likely not affect whether or not a biopsy is necessary, but it will help the patient realize that we carefully examined the lesion.

In describing the craft of magic, Henning Nelms wrote,

> As the object of the effect is to convince the spectators, their interpretation of the evidence is the only thing that counts. When the effect consists in taking a cannonball from an empty hat, the audience must believe that the hat is empty and that the cannonball is heavy. If the spectators accept this, a one-ounce half-globe of paper-mâché is as good as a twenty-pound iron sphere; if they regard the ball as an imitation, iron is no better than paper-mâché.
>
> (Nelms, 1969)

However, medicine is not magic. Whereas a magician does not need to produce an iron ball, doctors do need to make the right diagnosis and prescribe the right treatment. But if patients are not convinced of this, they will be left feeling as unsatisfied as the audience watching a magician who does produce an iron ball but does not convince the audience of it. Such dissatisfaction can lead to poor adherence and poor treatment outcomes. "Their interpretation of the evidence is the only thing that counts" is great wisdom when it comes to influencing the beliefs and behaviors of other people.

7.1.5 Timeliness

Showing up on time for clinic is *de rigueur*. Additionally, we must avoid looking at our watches when we are with patients. Looking at our watches during a visit with a patient might unintentionally communicate to the patient that we are in a hurry to leave and don't care about them. Instead, placing a clock on the wall directly behind where the patient sits allows us to look at the time while having the patient think we are looking at them and paying close attention.

7.2 Assessing Patients' Satisfaction

The easiest and most effective way to assess patients' satisfaction is to ask them for feedback directly, such as through surveys. They can tell us about the strengths of our office and identify areas for improvement. Positive reinforcement encourages us and our staff to continue the aspects of their visit that patients liked. If patients note aspects that they did not like, we should consider it a gift (which is not always easy to do!) and take advantage of their advice to improve the clinic experience for future patients. Patients may not be right about diagnostic or treatment issues, but they are always right about how they perceived things went.

Research from surveys reveals that the single most important factor that determines patients' satisfaction is whether or not they felt they saw a friendly, caring doctor (**Table 7.2**) (Uhas and Camacho, 2008). How long we keep patients waiting and how much time we spend with them in the examination room are statistically associated with patient satisfaction but only account for a small portion of the variation in satisfaction. Almost all the variation in overall patient satisfaction is determined by whether patients *perceive* that we are friendly, caring doctors. Satisfaction is not determined by how much we care (we care a lot!) but by patients' perceptions of how much we care.

There are many ways to conduct surveys. We can distribute a quick, one-page survey in the office ourselves. We can hire independent services to administer and analyze surveys or to call or write to patients. These approaches vary in their ease and cost. One particularly easy and inexpensive way to assess patient satisfaction is an online patient-satisfaction survey service, such as the now-defunct website www.DrScore.com, founded by one of this book's authors (**Figure 7.1**).

TABLE 7.2

Physician-Related Factors and Their Correlation with Patient Satisfaction

Factor	Correlation with Patient Satisfaction
Age	0.01
First visit	−0.03
Routine reason for visit	0.04
Male gender	−0.009
Waiting time	−0.13
Time spent with doctor	0.11
Caring attitude and friendliness	**0.87**

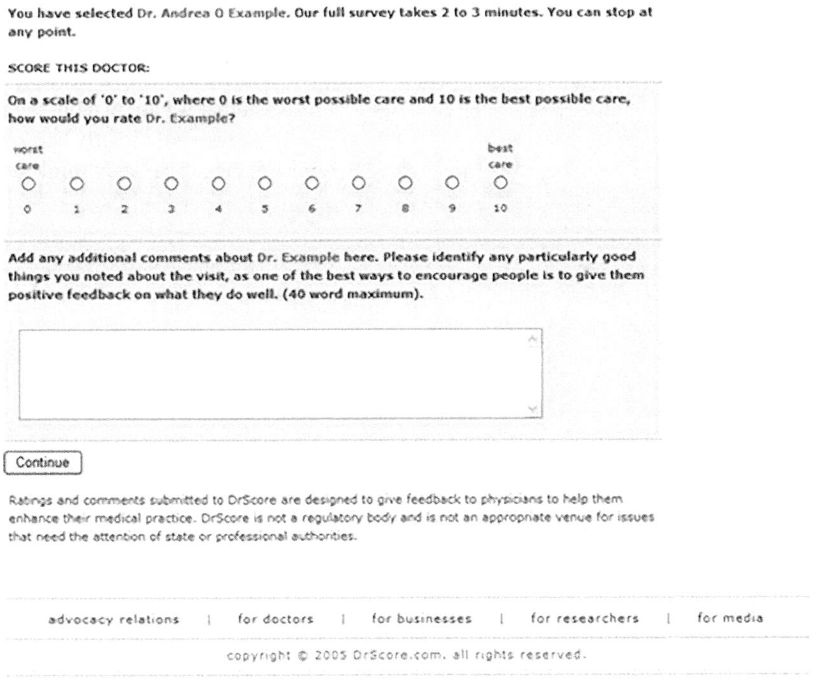

You have selected Dr. Andrea O Example. Our full survey takes 2 to 3 minutes. You can stop at any point.

SCORE THIS DOCTOR:

On a scale of '0' to '10', where 0 is the worst possible care and 10 is the best possible care, how would you rate Dr. Example?

worst care   best care

○ ○ ○ ○ ○ ○ ○ ○ ○ ○ ○
0   1   2   3   4   5   6   7   8   9   10

Add any additional comments about Dr. Example here. Please identify any particularly good things you noted about the visit, as one of the best ways to encourage people is to give them positive feedback on what they do well. (40 word maximum).

Continue

Ratings and comments submitted to DrScore are designed to give feedback to physicians to help them enhance their medical practice. DrScore is not a regulatory body and is not an appropriate venue for issues that need the attention of state or professional authorities.

advocacy relations | for doctors | for businesses | for researchers | for media

copyright © 2005 DrScore.com. all rights reserved.

FIGURE 7.1 **An example of an online patient satisfaction survey at the now-defunct website www.DrScore.com.** Online surveys are a cheap and easy way to assess patients' satisfaction.

TABLE 7.3

Patients' Comments on Their Experience with a Dermatologist

1	This was my first visit with [the doctor]. He was very thorough in examining me. Since I have a history of skin cancer, he asked me if I use sunscreen regularly and also asked if I have family members who have had skin cancer. Upon answering yes, he gave me two copies of recommended sunscreens. One for me and one for my sister who is not even a patient of his. This shows his great concern for everyone to help prevent skin cancer.
2	Excellent—I go to eight different doctors, but [these doctors] operate the friendliest, most efficient office. The nurses are all caring, efficient, and friendly.
3	I would have wished not to have been there so long. I got there 10 min early. 40 min after the appointment time, I went to the exam room to wait another 30-plus min. There must be some way to schedule appointments so wait time is not as long.
4	I got to see the doctor; he was patient, kind, and answered all my questions, even though it was for a different issue than when I had made the appt.
5	I was extremely impressed with his kind and concerned demeanor and the time he gave me. He checked me over thoroughly and spent time reviewing my melanoma on my face. I could not get over how kind he was! It was refreshing and gave me confidence in his care.
6	The exam was thorough, and the operative procedure was adequately explained. I never felt rushed.
7	He listens, cares, and is very good at what he does. I will remain with him as my doctor.
8	He made me feel comfortable when he first entered the room, and he made sure I understood what he was doing.
9	The staff was extremely courteous and friendly. It was a very pleasant experience.
10	He explains what he is doing and why; he also emphasizes how to protect against further problems.
11	He is friendly and very concerned about his patients.
12	[The doctor] gets a 10 out of 10 not just because he is a good doctor, but also because he spends time with me. He does not act rushed when I have questions and is not afraid of a little quiet pause while I absorb info or try to formulate a new question.
13	The office is incredibly professional, pleasant, calm, and well-run. The staff is very nice and helpful. I felt I was in good hands. It was the best doctor's office experience I have ever had! Thanks for not having a TV in the lobby, but a fountain instead.
14	He took his time to explain his answer properly when I asked a question. He also was looking at me as a person and did identify other issues with me that needed treatment. I would recommend him to other people. Thanks.
15	His examination was thorough and candid. He did not rush me through the exam; he was methodical, took the time to explain the condition, and recommended treatment. A welcome break from the assembly line appointments administered by most doctors these days.
16	I have appreciated his conservatism and calm manner as I have visited him over the past eight years or so. He has always given me excellent and timely care.
17	[The doctor] is one of the finest physicians I have ever encountered regardless of specialty. His bedside manner and thoroughness are outstanding. . . . [H]e is to be commended both as a caregiver and a technically wonderful physician. 10 out of 10, the best.

18	He was very good with all the questions that I asked him. He told me what he was going to do before he did it; this is one of the best visits that I have ever had with a doctor. We needed more doctors like [him].
19	It is too bad there are not more doctors that care about their patients as much as he does! I wish I had gone to see him before the ER visits and family physician visit. His office is beautiful!
20	[The doctor] was very through and explained the proper care and prevention and was not in any hurry.
21	Both [the doctor] and his assistant . . . were courteous, informative, and professional.

Source: Collected from www.DrScore.com.

The open comments from patient surveys demonstrate what patients prioritize in their physicians. A dermatologist from Kentucky shared the open comments patients made about him on a DrScore.com survey (**Table 7.3**). Notice that the comments focus far more on friendliness, caring, and bedside manner—which patients can easily judge—than on technical expertise—which is more difficult for patients to assess. Notice that the third comment in Table 7.3 is from a patient who waited a long time—over one hour!—to be seen by the doctor. Yet this patient nevertheless rated their visit a 10 out of 10. Patients may not like waiting, but most will gladly do so to spend time with someone they perceive to be a caring doctor.

When patients develop positive perceptions of us, they will trust the treatments we prescribe. Indeed, they will not be as scared about the potential side effects they see on the package insert inside their medication box. They will use their medication correctly, and their conditions will improve. They will also be far more open to the idea of trying a novel medication because we have built a relationship of trust over time. They will also be satisfied with their care, and this outcome alone should make our efforts worthwhile.

8

Setting the Right Office Visit Context

8.1 The Halo Effect

The halo effect is the tendency for one attribute of a person or object to "spill over" and affect perceptions of other, even unrelated attributes of that person or object (Davis and Feldman, 2014). For example, attractive people are generally viewed as more intelligent and trustworthy than less attractive people. Attractive individuals receive better grades than unattractive people of the same intelligence and are treated more leniently by the judicial system. In this example, attractiveness confers a "halo" that positively affects people's perceptions of the individual's other attributes.

We can apply the halo effect to promote patient satisfaction. Since most patients are not equipped to assess our clinical skills accurately, they judge us based on our overall appearance and bedside manner. Imagine one clinic with a clean, organized waiting room that offers complimentary coffee, a variety of magazines, courteous staff at the front desk, kind nurses, and a physician wearing a freshly ironed, immaculate white coat. Now imagine another clinic with rude staff, an untidy waiting room, and a disheveled, poorly dressed physician. Although the physician in the second clinic might be highly competent, patients may make judgments based on the poor appearance of the clinic setting and conclude that this office offers substandard care.

8.2 The Blue Vein Illusion and the Power of Context

The power of context to affect our perceptions is illustrated by the apparently blue color of veins (Feldman, 2008). We should know that veins are not blue from "deoxygenated hemoglobin" because we know that blood is red when we draw it from veins. Our veins cannot be blue. But even knowing that veins cannot be blue and knowing it is only an optical illusion, if we look at our veins, the veins still appear blue (**Figure 8.1**). We cannot control the power that context has on our perceptions.

DOI: 10.1201/9781003367628-10

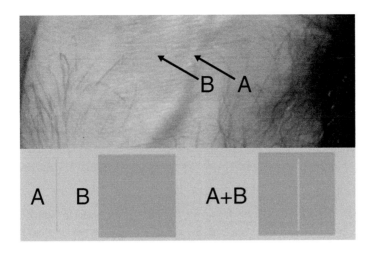

FIGURE 8.1 **The blue vein illusion.** In this figure, line A is the color of the vein, and it is clearly not blue. Square B is the color of the surrounding skin. When line A is seen in the context of square B, the line has a bluish appearance.

8.3 Context of the Office Visit

Setting the right context—maintaining a clean, neatly arranged office; having staff who are friendly and attentive; posting office signs that convey caring and trust; and adhering to a schedule in which patients are seen on time—helps ensure that our patients perceive we care about them. They might even be more willing to overlook negative aspects of their visit if the appearance of our clinic gives the clear impression that we care about them.

One common scenario is that patients might arrive at our office thinking that doctors only care about money. This perception might be reinforced by signs at the reception desk that outline copayment policies, returned check policies, and accepted credit cards (**Figure 8.2**). Ideally, our office attributes should not be set up to reinforce such biases.

In place of too many signs about our offices' financial expectations, we might post a sign that reads, "We appreciate the trust you put in us and are proud to provide you medical care of the highest quality."

Other strategies to convey the right message to our patients and improve the atmosphere of our clinic are outlined in Section 8.4 in a checklist format that facilitates audits of the office environment (Rajpara, 2012).

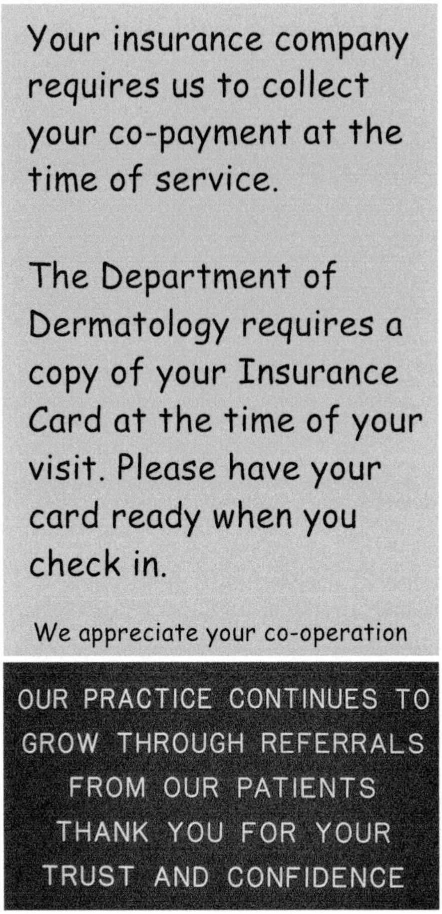

Your insurance company requires us to collect your co-payment at the time of service.

The Department of Dermatology requires a copy of your Insurance Card at the time of your visit. Please have your card ready when you check in.

We appreciate your co-operation

OUR PRACTICE CONTINUES TO GROW THROUGH REFERRALS FROM OUR PATIENTS THANK YOU FOR YOUR TRUST AND CONFIDENCE

FIGURE 8.2 Office signs. One of these signs provides information on important office policies while the other does not. Which one will give the patient the impression that we care more about our patients than about money?

8.4 Office Evaluation Checklist

(Reproduced with permission from *The Dermatologist*.)

8.4.1 Waiting Room

1. Magazines are in good condition.
2. Water and cup dispenser is clean.
3. The trash can is not next to the water dispenser.
4. Ceiling panels are unstained.

5. The check-in desk is in good condition.
6. Patient fliers are on a bulletin board, not taped to windows.
7. All windowsills are clean.

8.4.2 Clinic Hallways

1. Entrance door is well maintained.
2. Nurses' desk is well maintained.
3. Nurses' area is clean.
4. Patient folders are in good condition.
5. Wallpaper is well maintained.
6. No papers are taped to walls or doors.
7. All signs are laminated.
8. Exam room doors are clean.
9. Cryoablation device is not easily accessible to patients.
10. Chart holders on the examination room doors are clean.
11. Dry erase boards outside patient rooms are clean.
12. Pictures and frames are in good condition.
13. Hallways are generally clean and free of dust.
14. There are no scuff marks on the floors.

8.4.3 Exam Room

1. Wallpaper is well maintained.
2. There are no holes in the walls.
3. There is no writing on the walls.
4. There is no tape left on the walls.
5. No nails are showing in the wall.
6. Plastic information and folder holders are clean.
7. Sinks are clean.
8. Mirrors are clean.
9. Patient chair and footstool are clean.
10. Equipment tray is clean or covered with a clean drape.
11. Trash cans are well maintained.
12. Patient and visitor chairs are well maintained.
13. Coat hangers are well maintained.
14. Doorknobs are clean.
15. All cabinets are well maintained.
16. All windowsills are clean.
17. Floors are clean.

9

Fostering Patient Accountability

Like trust, accountability is at the foundation of getting patients to use medication. Accountability may be the single most underappreciated, critical component to getting patients to take their medication. Creating greater accountability may also represent low-hanging fruit for improving our patients' treatment adherence and outcomes.

Accountability is a widely used motivational technique, be it through formal accounting of sales in business or reporting research progress at weekly laboratory meetings. While there are many reasons patients are not able to take their medication, fostering accountability can improve patient adherence regardless of the reasons for poor adherence.

We can hold our patients accountable in a number of ways. If we establish a strong physician–patient relationship, our patients will naturally want to please us; they will want to use their medication to avoid letting us down. We can also schedule regular follow-up visits to make them accountable for using their medication in anticipation of their office visits.

To prove the importance of accountability, let us examine the parable of the piano teacher.

9.1 Parable of the Piano Teacher

A piano teacher gave her students sheet music, told them to practice every day, and held weekly lessons with her students for eight to twelve weeks, after which time she held a piano recital at which all the students performed. The audience loved the music; all the children sounded terrific. They performed well at the recital because they had practiced at least some each week leading up to the recital.

Another piano teacher, straight out of piano teacher school, thought that the weekly visits were a very inefficient strategy. He realized that it was the students' practicing, rather than the weekly piano lesson visits, that had made the children play so well. So, he gave his students sheet music and told them, "We are going to hold our recital in eight to twelve weeks, but we are going to forgo the weekly lessons. What makes you play well is practicing at home, not the lessons. Just practice every day, and I will see you again at the recital."

This recital, though, sounded execrable. Without the weekly lessons to encourage the students to practice on their own, they did not practice much at all until just days before the recital (**Figure 9.1**).

Now, what if the second piano teacher said, "Ooh, that recital was terrible. The students aren't practicing as they should. I'll go to the medical literature and see

DOI: 10.1201/9781003367628-11

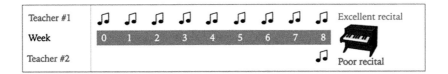

FIGURE 9.1 **Comparison of two different piano teachers in preparation for a recital in eight weeks.** Teacher #1 holds weekly piano lessons, whereas teacher #2 instructs students to practice weekly at home. Predictably, the recital led by teacher #1 sounds incomparably better as the weekly lessons encouraged students to practice each week, as indicated by the music notes. On the other hand, the students led by teacher #2 hardly practiced at all until just before the recital.

what doctors do to get patients to take their medicine. I'll do motivational interviewing, address the cost of treatment, keep the recommended music simple, give the students written instructions, and have them use a reminder system, but we won't need weekly lessons because it's the practice, not the lessons, that make people play piano well." Would the recital sound any better? Not likely. The anticipation of the weekly lessons is critically important in holding the piano students accountable for practicing.

9.2 School or Work Assignments

No one, not in any field of human activity, gives a person a new assignment and says, "Work on this project every day. I will meet with you again in eight to twelve weeks." Well, no one except us doctors. No research lab director would say to a bright, industrious student on a summer research rotation, even a highly motivated one who desires a dermatology residency position, "Here is your project. Work on it every day, and we will meet again at the end of the summer." Even highly motivated, exceptionally effective medical students would likely fail to accomplish much in such a circumstance. The only people who take such an approach to getting people to do something are doctors. (And our patients are typically not as high functioning, industrious, and motivated as students who want to get into dermatology!)

HELPFUL HINT: CANCELLING A WEEKLY TEAM MEETING

Dr. Feldman's research team meets once a week, at noon on Fridays, at which time they discuss the progress on their projects. If the lab director was called on Monday, was asked to give a lecture out of town on Friday, and accepted the invitation, on what day should he let his minions know that the Friday lab meeting is cancelled? He could tell them on Monday; if he did, his minions might not work very hard that week (adversely affecting their chances of getting a dermatology residency spot). On the other hand, if he let the minions know on Thursday night or Friday morning that he was cancelling the meeting, the minions would get in their usual full week of work. Because he cares so much about them and their success, he waits until the last minute to let them know. Note that it is not the meeting that causes them to work; it is the expectation that there will be a meeting that drives their behavior. Similarly, the expectation that the patient will report their progress to the physician strongly motivates patients to fill their prescription, start the treatment, and use it well.

The way we practice—the standard way we start patients on a new medication—is set up to fail. Giving patients a medication and telling them, "See you in eight to twelve weeks" does not make sense at all. Now, we are not exactly like the piano teacher who gives kids sheet music and says, "Practice every day; see you in eight to twelve weeks." No, we are far worse! We are more like a piano teacher who says, "Here is a prescription for some sheet music. Take it to the sheet music store. I do not have any idea how much the sheet music will cost you, whether your insurance will pay for it, or how much hassle and paperwork will be required to obtain reimbursement from the insurer. But get the sheet music and practice every day. By the way, practicing may cause a rash, headache, diarrhea, or possibly a serious infection. But practice every day, and I will see you at the recital in eight to twelve weeks. And if the recital doesn't sound good, which it often doesn't, I will give you one or two new, more costly musical instruments to practice at the same time."

Is there any doubt that our standard approach to getting patients to use medications is lacking?

9.3 Clinical Trials versus Real-Life Practice

Clinical trials designed to assess drug efficacy are different from clinical practice. Drugs that work very well in clinical trials may not work as well in clinical practice; one of our mentors taught us, "When new drugs are approved, use them fast, before they stop working."

Clinical trials demonstrate how effectively and how quickly a drug works; statistically significant improvements in outcomes may be seen as early as one to two weeks after beginning the drug. The publications describing the clinical trial results display elegant curves with data points every two weeks and illustrate how the drug continues to yield improvements over eight to twelve weeks or longer. The Food and Drug Administration approves the drug, and the package insert describes how well it is tolerated and how patients exhibit disease improvement in eight to twelve weeks.

Once the drug hits the market, we may prescribe it and tell patients to return in eight to twelve weeks. That's not what they did in the study! All those interim study visits in the trial drive patients to use their treatment (like a visit to the dentist promotes flossing); all the monitoring in the study and treatment diaries encourage better use, not to mention that we don't have to worry in clinical trials that patients won't fill the prescription (**Figure 9.2**). In real-life practice, since there is

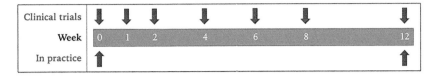

FIGURE 9.2 **The frequency of office visits in clinical trials greatly differs from that seen in clinical practice.** Clinical trials typically include frequent assessment visits. Visits at baseline (week zero) and weeks one, two, four, six, eight, and twelve are common. These visits allow researchers to assess the drug's effectiveness over the course of treatment. On the other hand, in the real world, visits typically occur every twelve weeks. Much like the Heisenberg uncertainty principle in physics, which states that measuring the momentum or position of a particle changes its momentum or position, the office visits done to assess efficacy in a clinical trial change the effectiveness of the drug, making the drug more effective by improving adherence to the treatment.

no follow-up between writing the prescription and seeing the patient back at the eight-to-twelve-week follow-up visit, patients don't use the drug well and don't see good efficacy. They often return reporting that the drug did not work or that they had stopped using it because they developed some side effects that they could not tolerate for eight to twelve weeks.

Instead, we can have our patients return for a follow-up visit (or arrange some other form of contact) shortly after initiating treatment, much as we do in clinical trials. The higher frequency of office visits in clinical trials indirectly increases adherence, so we can use a similar strategy to improve adherence in real-life clinical practice. While frequent follow-up visits might not be practical, scheduling the first return visit at week one instead of at week eight may be practical. Approaches other than a return visit—even a planned phone call one week after starting treatment—may be suitable alternatives.

9.4 White Coat Compliance

Mothers of children with acne often tell us, "Doctor, it is so frustrating. You always catch it on a good day. You do not see what it is normally like." Their children's acne is better when they visit us. The reason we seem to catch patients on a good day is the same reason we do not use blood glucose levels to assess control of diabetes at office visits; patients use their medication much better in the few days preceding the visit. Similarly, just as individuals tend to floss their teeth more often prior to visiting the dentist, our patients use their medications just before they come to see us (Feldman and Camacho, 2007).

When this concept was presented to a neurologist who had specialized in treating Parkinson's disease for over eight years, she explained, "Every day in clinic, the spouses tell me, 'Doctor, it is so frustrating. When you examine him, he moves just fine. But when he is at home, he can barely move at all.'" The neurologist had thought the stress of the examination was somehow altering her patients' neurotransmitters; more likely, the patients simply started taking their medication in anticipation of the visit.

We can use this phenomenon, known as white coat compliance, to hold our patients accountable by scheduling a follow-up visit shortly after starting a new treatment to assess how well the treatment is working (and thereby improve adherence and how well the treatment is working). Dr. Lawrence Feldman, formerly of Westminster, Maryland, described how the concept of white coat compliance changed the way he treated acne. Instead of scheduling return visits in six to eight weeks, he had patients come back in two weeks and saw better results.

9.4.1 "Cyber White Coat Compliance"

While accountability is a social phenomenon, it does not necessarily require direct human contact. For example, in one study, a web-based, weekly reporting intervention doubled adherence to acne treatment in adolescents (Yentzer and Gosnell, 2011). Such weekly reporting instills a sense of accountability—essentially, cyber or digital white coat compliance. Digital approaches designed to mimic human interaction and social pressure may be a low-cost, highly feasible way to generate the accountability needed to get patients to use treatment. Therefore, if frequent appointments are unfeasible, we ask our patients to call or email us in a few days or, at most, a week to report how the medication is working, which provides a similar social pressure of accountability.

9.5 A Nobel Peace Prize Example

In 2006, Muhammad Yunus and Grameen Bank were awarded the Nobel Peace Prize for their use of microlending to "create economic and social development from below." Grameen Bank, founded by Yunus, issues small loans to poor people on favorable terms. The steps to lift people out of poverty, according to Yunus, are to lend them money in amounts that suit them and teach them basic financial principles. Loans may be for as little as $25, although the mean is $200. People can use the loans to purchase a cell phone, chicken, or cow, providing a basis for a small business: a pay phone operation, eggs for sale, or milk to sell. Loan repayment rates are in excess of 98%, far better than with traditional lending! Microcredit is viewed as a very promising way to get people out of poverty.

Is merely giving poor people access to microcredit the solution to poverty? Giving them a loan may be necessary, but it alone is insufficient. The program at Grameen Bank involves more than just making small loans. The program also brings together groups of five women who already know each other who develop business plans and *meet weekly* with a bank representative to discuss their business development, marketing, and sales efforts. There is enormous social pressure within these groups to market effectively, work to sell products, and repay the loans. The accountability of these women to each other and the accountability provided by the weekly meetings at which the women must present what they've done to sell their product over the past week may be just as important to the success of the program as the loan money itself, just as accountability to the physician may be as important as the prescription for getting patients well.

Section 3

Practicality—Simplicity and Education

DOI: 10.1201/9781003367628-12

10

Involving Patients in the Choice of Treatment

Involving patients in the choice of treatment is important because patients often have strong preferences for certain therapies, and those preferences may be different from ours. Typically, the various treatment options for a given dermatologic condition exhibit a wide spectrum in terms of efficacy, safety, and convenience. Some of these issues may be of utmost importance to one patient and of little consequence to another. Some patients prefer a medication that acts rapidly and care little about potential side effects. Others are risk averse and would rather err on the side of safety. Doctors are often older, married, and not suffering acutely as the patient is and thus may not feel the same need for rapid improvement and risk-taking that an unmarried patient might feel when thinking the rash prevents them from dating. Sometimes, otherwise rational patients may display a strong aversion to a particular drug or side effect based on their past experience or the experience of a friend, a very powerful phenomenon that we can use to help patients. We discuss this topic further in Chapter 15: Giving Salient Descriptions.

Patients also differ in how skin disease affects them. A treatment that we view as safe and appropriate might seem far too risky to some patients. Others might deem the same therapy inadequately aggressive. Furthermore, one patient might do anything to avoid a needle (we have ways of dealing with this fear; see Chapter 14: Anchoring), while another might believe an injection is just what they need. Patients' preferences can be wildly unpredictable, but they keep our practices interesting.

10.1 The Ikea Effect

The Ikea effect holds that when we put work into obtaining or building something personally, we value it more highly (Davis and Feldman, 2014). The namesake example is that a piece of furniture from Ikea, which typically requires self-assembly, holds more value than an identical item that comes pre-assembled.

The Ikea effect suggests that when patients are involved in their treatment plans—when they are making decisions and working with us to solve problems—they become more invested in improving their own health. We can utilize several strategies to facilitate this sort of involvement. One approach is to frame treatment options in a way that the patient adopts the treatment plan as their own idea. For instance, we can begin with the open-ended question: "What is important to you in a treatment?" If the patient has difficulty responding, we can progress to a more

 DOI: 10.1201/9781003367628-13

specific question, allowing the patient to choose from multiple options: "Do you prefer a treatment that gets rid of your symptoms as quickly as possible or one that works slower but has fewer side effects?" By facilitating and engaging patients in this dialogue, we can engender a sense of responsibility to adhere to the treatment regimen. This feeling of ownership only becomes possible when the treatment plan is no longer our idea but theirs.

RECOMMENDED QUOTE

We can involve patients in selecting a treatment by asking, "What is important to you in a treatment?" An appropriate follow-up question is, "Do you prefer a treatment that gets rid of your symptoms as quickly as possible or one that works slower but has fewer side effects?"

10.2 Topical Treatments: Choosing a Vehicle

The age-old dogma for treating skin lesions is "If it is wet, dry it; if it is dry, wet it." We were indoctrinated that conditions that produce dry, scaly lesions should be treated with ointments. We were taught that ointments are inherently more potent than less occlusive vehicles such as creams or lotions because ointments deliver more of the active drug by increasing skin penetration. We were taught to encourage patients with psoriasis and atopic dermatitis to use ointments, even when they are reluctant to do so.

This way of thinking did have some underlying scientific rationale. Many years ago, most ointments did deliver higher amounts of the drug into the skin than did creams or lotions. The occlusive properties of some ointments increase epidermal hydration and reduce barrier function, thereby increasing drug penetration. There may even be anti-inflammatory effects associated with improving epidermal barrier function using an occlusive agent. Nevertheless, patients will not realize these beneficial effects if they do not apply the product.

Newer non-ointment preparations, though, are designed to deliver the drug without occluding the skin. Moreover, diseased skin has poor barrier function, so the occlusive properties of an ointment may not be needed. While moisturizing the skin and repairing the epidermal barrier may confer anti-inflammatory effects, they are not essential for controlling inflammation or making skin lesions resolve. Systemic drugs such as cyclosporine and infliximab exert powerful anti-inflammatory effects and can completely clear psoriatic plaques, yet they do not moisturize the skin. Clobetasol, an even more potent anti-inflammatory agent, does not need to be applied in a messy, occlusive vehicle to be effective.

One common method of measuring the potency of a topical corticosteroid is the vasoconstrictor assay. This assay measures the amount of blanching that occurs when the agent is applied; the stronger the steroid, the greater the blanching. The assay assesses two of the three factors that determine the potency of a topical steroid: (1) how potent the drug is in activating corticosteroid receptors and (2) how well the vehicle delivers the drug into the skin. However, the vasoconstrictor assay does not assess a third, often-overlooked factor that affects the potency of topical steroid preparations: whether patients will apply the medication. A messy product that demonstrates a high potency in the laboratory setting does not necessarily work well in patients who will not apply a messy product.

Poor adherence has a dramatic effect on the efficacy of topical agents. Steroid ointments, which may be wonderfully potent under the controlled conditions of the vasoconstrictor assay, may show minimal potency in real-life patients who dislike the greasy feeling of an ointment preparation (**Figure 10.1**).

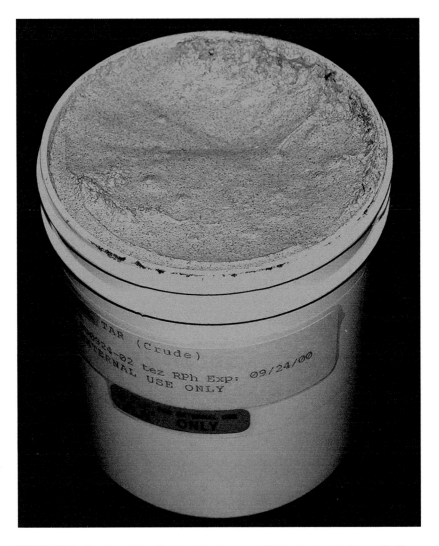

FIGURE 10.1   Crude coal tar. Crude coal tar is a very effective treatment when applied in an office or hospital setting, but it is far too messy for most patients to use at home. Ointments pose similar issues in many patients.

Fortunately, one of the major advancements in the care of patients with psoriasis was the development of a host of vehicle options for delivering steroids topically. We still have ointments for patients who prefer them, and some patients do like them as ointments soften hard scale, reduce the pain of fissures, and make scale disappear immediately (the scale does not go away; the change in refraction merely makes it transparent). We now also have creams, foams, gels, lotions, shampoos, sprays, and tapes. For each patient, one of these vehicles will be the best. Which one? The one they will use.

Housman and colleagues studied the characteristics of topical vehicles that affect patients' preferences for various vehicles (Housman, 2002). Seven characteristics mattered: ease of application, time required for application, absorption, how it feels to touch, how it smells, how it feels on the skin, and how much it stains. Patients with psoriasis were asked to rate a variety of vehicles—creams, foams, gels, ointments, and solutions—using these criteria. Overall, they preferred the less messy products, particularly foams and solutions, over the more moisturizing vehicles such as ointments.

The notion that patients find ointments messy is not new. Patients have been complaining about ointments for years. Aversion to ointments may explain why so many prescriptions for psoriasis medications went unfilled in Denmark (Storm and Anderson, 2008). One approach that has been suggested is to give patients a less messy product to use during the day and an ointment to apply at night, when patients presumably do not mind using the ointment. But when patients were asked to characterize their daytime and nighttime preferences for different vehicles, no significant differences were observed (Housman, 2002). In other words, patients generally did not like using the ointment, either during the day or at night (**Figure 10.2**).

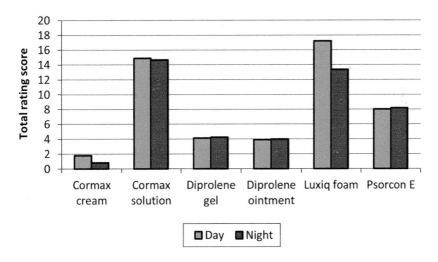

FIGURE 10.2 Patients daytime and nighttime preferences for various vehicles. Patients strongly preferred using foams and solutions over creams and ointments, regardless of the time of day.

Many patients seem to prefer the new "lighter" vehicles like the foam. However, other than asking patients directly, there is no *a priori* way to predict what vehicle will be best for a given patient. Ideally, if samples are available, we might have the patient try different vehicles and see which one they prefer. While we have been taught that ointments are best for dry, scaly conditions, this is simply not true; if you are not yet convinced of this fact, it may be good to jump ahead to Chapter 24: Skin Cap for Psoriasis. The best vehicle for a particular patient is usually the vehicle they will use.

10.3 The Default Option

In research survey studies, patients say they want to know about their options and participate in treatment planning. But in the clinic, patients often ask for clear guidance from us on what treatment to take; they value our opinion about which treatment is best. While we should involve patients in the choice of treatment, we should also guide them, rather than giving them an array of options with no input at all. So many treatment options are available that patients may have difficulty knowing which one to choose. In fact, they may even hesitate to choose any treatment at all, prolonging their suffering with undertreated disease.

Behavioral scientists studying employees' retirement plans have found that many employees do not sign up for a retirement savings plan, even when employers gave the employees free money in the form of matching funds. This dynamic left many employees without an adequate retirement plan. To address the problem, employers began offering employees more retirement plan options. Providing more savings options was counterproductive, causing more employees to forgo making any retirement contributions! The more complicated the choice, the more employees did not bother to check the box to sign up for retirement savings. Instead, they went with the default option, which was not to sign up at all.

The solution for getting employees to participate was simple: make participating in a basic retirement plan the default option unless the employee had chosen some other plan (or no plan at all). We can use the default option to help patients select and adhere to a single therapy. We can tell them, "The standard approach is drug A, but you could also choose from among drugs X, Y, and Z if you prefer." If we wish to encourage patients to select drug A because we think it is the most appropriate, we might tell them, "In this situation, the standard approach is drug A, but you have dozens of other choices. Let me get a few books for you to read that describe these other options in detail." Patients are not going to want to read those books. The more difficult, complicated, and time consuming we make it to choose another approach, the more likely patients will go along with the default plan that we suggest. If we want to nudge patients further toward the plan we think is best, we can add, "I had a patient whose disease was a lot like yours, and they did well on drug A." We will further discuss the value of such anecdotes in Chapter 15: Giving Salient Descriptions.

RECOMMENDED QUOTE

We can help patients choose the best treatment among many options by stating, "In this situation, the standard approach is drug A, but you have dozens of other choices. Let me get a few books for you to read that describe these other options in detail."

11

Reducing the Burden of Treatment

We should strive to make treatment as easy as possible for our patients and not create needless hurdles. Patients already experience the burden of their disease and are busy with their lives. We should avoid treatments that are worse than the disease. We should also avoid complicated approaches that patients will not have time to do. Reducing the burden of treatment helps promote adherence and can be achieved via a variety of strategies, such as prescribing combination drugs, minimizing complexity, and shortening the treatment interval.

11.1 Using Combination Drugs

Sometimes we want patients to take more than one medication to benefit from multiple mechanisms of action to treat their disease. But giving patients multiple treatments creates a hurdle to adherence. When more prescriptions are given, fewer prescriptions are used. The more complicated the treatment, the less patients follow the treatment regimen. One helpful approach, commonly used in treating acne or psoriasis, is to prescribe a product that combines two or more medications. In treating acne, we often want patients to use an antiseptic product (perhaps benzoyl peroxide) along with a topical retinoid (such as adapalene). But it is hard enough getting patients with acne to apply a single product on a regular basis. Giving patients more than one product to use complicates the regimen and makes adherence more challenging. In one study, when patients were given one, two, or three or more different prescriptions to fill, 9%, 40%, and 31%, respectively, did not even fill all their prescriptions (Anderson, 2015). Giving patients multiple prescriptions reduces primary adherence.

HELPFUL HINT: SYNCING REFILLS

Even going to the pharmacy to pick up refills represents a barrier to adherence. When patients are on multiple medications, their prescriptions may be out of sync, requiring multiple calls and visits to the pharmacy each month to get refills. This issue is a needless hurdle. Pharmacists can give patients a few extra pills or whatever is needed to get all the prescriptions synced up so that they can be filled at the same time. Use of a mail order pharmacy is another approach to help minimize the burden of being on chronic medical treatment.

DOI: 10.1201/9781003367628-14

Another study found that secondary adherence is higher when patients are given a single product with two active ingredients than when they receive two separate products (Yentzer and Ade, 2010). Prescribing a product that contains two active agents—such as Epiduo or Epiduo Forte (benzoyl peroxide/adapaline), Benzaclin (clindamycin/benzoyl peroxide), or Veltin (clindamycin/tretinoin)—makes treating acne less complicated and may improve patients' adherence.

In treating psoriasis, Dovonex (calcipotriene) ointment works too slowly by itself and thus is best used in combination with a topical steroid. Sequential treatment regimens—initially using both drugs daily, then one on weekdays and the other on weekends, and then one for maintenance—represent an alternative but are overly complicated. Applying two medications at different times of the day increases the chance that patients will miss doses. Moreover, applying them simultaneously might dilute them, potentially reducing their efficacy. A combination product such as Dovobet, Taclonex, Enstilar, or Wynzora (calcipotriene/betamethasone dipropionate) or Duobrii (tazarotene/halobetasol) is useful in this situation. By giving our patients both drugs in a single container for once-daily use, we can make topical therapy for psoriasis less complex and adherence more likely.

11.2 Simplifying the Treatment Regimen

When patients present with refractory skin conditions, we might be eager to add different types of medications, switch to more potent medications, or institute measures that promote occlusion and penetration. Recognizing that treatment failures in dermatology often result from poor adherence, we can see how these efforts might be counterproductive. The solution is not to make the treatment regimen more complicated but to make it less complex.

For example, consider a child whose atopic dermatitis is refractory to emollients and various topical steroids. Adding stronger steroids, oral antihistamines, and wet wraps only makes it more difficult for the parents and child to adhere to treatment. A more reasonable approach would be to limit treatment to a single topical steroid and focus on using that one treatment well. By eliminating ancillary medications, the family can concentrate on applying the one steroid properly, and the child's lesions will clear beautifully in a few days, much as they would if they were treated in the hospital.

We also tend to make the treatment of psoriasis more complicated than necessary. Dermatology textbooks recommend keratinolytic agents such as salicylic acid for breaking up psoriatic scales and enhancing the penetration of topical steroids. *Rook's Textbook of Dermatology* claims, "Even the most potent steroid is useless if painted on the surface of thickly heaped-up psoriasis" (Burns and Breathnach, 2010). Similarly, Habif's *Clinical Dermatology: A Color Guide to Diagnosis and Therapy* states that "scale must be removed first to facilitate penetration of medicine" (Habif, 2009). These recommendations, though, contradict the results of studies indicating that diseased skin—even if thick and scaly—exhibits poor barrier function. Furthermore, in numerous clinical trials topical clobetasol alone—without any descaling agent—was highly effective in clearing thick, scaly psoriatic plaques.

Salicylic acid remains a useful agent to reduce hyperkeratosis but is not necessary for permitting steroid penetration, reducing inflammation, or clearing psoriatic plaques. If we can motivate our patients to use their topical steroids, their
lesions will improve. Making the regimen more complex by giving separate keratolytic agents may reduce adherence, making the disease more "resistant" to treatment. Perhaps *Rook's Textbook of Dermatology* would have been more accurate if
it read, "Even the most potent steroid is useless if it is not applied." For more on this
principle, see Chapter 25: Coral Reef Psoriasis.

11.3 Shortening the Treatment Time Horizon

For alcoholics, the heavy burden of quitting alcohol for the rest of their lives is
enough to drive them to drink. For this reason, the focus of Alcoholics Anonymous
is not on quitting forever, but rather on quitting for a single day—just one day. If the
alcoholic can accomplish this goal and do so consistently, then they have essentially
quit forever. The task of avoiding alcohol for a single day, one day at a time, appears
far less burdensome than quitting forever. Adhering to treatment for chronic skin
diseases is not altogether different.

One of the most effective methods of improving adherence is to begin with a
short treatment interval. Suggesting that patients use a medication, especially a topical one, several times a day for six to eight weeks will leave patients feeling that
the treatment is an extraordinary burden. Imagine being faced with the prospect
of applying a topical agent to lesions scattered throughout your body twice a day
for six to eight weeks. Imagine how difficult this task sounds, as busy as you are
already. Now imagine how much worse it would be if you were a parent in charge of
applying the medication to your child's skin for those six to eight weeks.

Now consider instead how you would interpret the burden if the doctor had
explained, "I am going to ask you to do something very difficult. I would like you to
apply the medication to the spots on your skin twice a day. But it is only for the next
three days. Then we will see you back in the office and gauge your improvement."
Patients will use the medication much better, will have witnessed the benefits of the
medication, will have developed a habit of using the medication, and will continue
therapy thereafter. In essence, shortening the treatment time horizon lets them see
the light at the end of the tunnel. It is a motivating force that strengthens their ability to bear the burden of treatment more easily.

RECOMMENDED QUOTE

An effective way to shorten the treatment time horizon is by explaining,
"I am going to ask you to do something very difficult. I would like you to
apply the medication to the spots on your skin twice a day. But it is only for
the next three days. Then we will see you back in the office and gauge your
improvement."

11.4 Switching to an Easier Treatment Regimen

The human brain is not designed to perceive reality in isolation; it is designed to appreciate contrasts. Our perceptions tend to be relative rather than absolute. A sweet cola product, for instance, may taste bitter if we drink it while eating ice cream. A 50°F day might seem warm during the dead of winter but would feel unusually cold during the summer. Our perceptions of touch, sight, smell, and sound are all affected by context.

So, too, are our perceptions of the burden of treatment. If we prescribe our patients a treatment regimen easier than their previous one, they might view their new regimen favorably. We might achieve this end by prescribing a single medication instead of two or switching to home phototherapy instead of office-based phototherapy. Applying a topical medication once a day is not easy, but it might seem easy to patients who were trying to do so twice a day. Similarly, using a topical spray is more difficult than taking a pill, but using the spray might seem effortless to patients who had previously been using an ointment.

To make a certain regimen seem easier, patients do not even need to have tried a more difficult treatment. Simply describing some arbitrary, more difficult treatment may be all that is required. We discuss this further in Chapter 14: Anchoring.

11.5 Selecting a Fast-Acting Agent

Positive feedback is a strong motivator—when patients see that their medication works, they will be motivated to continue using it. Therefore, a fast-acting agent may be more effective than a slow-acting one. We have a very short window after we prescribe a medication during which our patients adhere to the treatment regimen. Most patients will not patiently wait to see if a slow-acting medication works before they give up on it. When prescribing a slow-acting agent, such as Plaquenil (hydroxychloroquine) for lupus erythematosus, we advise initially pairing it with a fast-acting agent (for example, topical clobetasol) so that patients see rapid improvement in their disease and are encouraged to continue taking their medications.

11.6 Minimizing Costs of Treatment

Prescribing a medication patients cannot afford is not a sensible way to encourage adherence. We should prescribe low-cost equivalent medications when available, unless our patients specifically prefer a more expensive product. We can also use our electronic medical record system to auto-populate the following instructions for the pharmacist on our prescriptions: "If the pharmacy offers a similar but less expensive option, feel free to switch to that medication, if the patient wants to. Call me if there's any question." Even generic topical steroids can be very expensive. If we prescribe clobetasol but the pharmacy offers betamethasone at a lower price, if we and the patient are comfortable with that change, then we can have the pharmacist make the substitution.

RECOMMENDED QUOTE

To minimize the costs of treatment, we can use the following in the instructions for the pharmacist that appear on our prescriptions: "If the pharmacy offers a similar but less expensive option, feel free to switch to that medication, if the patient wants to. Call me if there's any question."

12

Educating and Providing Instructions

It is always a good idea to educate patients about their diagnosis and their medication. Do they know why they were given their medication and how they are supposed to use it? If they understand their disease and how to use the medication, they will be more likely to abide by our recommended treatment plan. To this end, providing patients with information about their condition and clear instructions for their treatment is critical for maximizing adherence.

Although this information seems basic, it does not always get transmitted to patients. One study conducted in Denmark looked at how often physicians gave patients basic information about the medication they prescribed at the same visit (Storm and Benfeldt, 2009). Shockingly, only two out of three patients were given the diagnosis or told the treatment duration. Only one in four patients were told the effect of the medication, and none were told the potential adverse effects or the cost of the medication. And even when patients were given this information, it was often presented in a way that was not effective. When patients were queried two weeks after the visit, most did not know the diagnosis, the duration of treatment, or how much of the medication to use. We could blame patients for not remembering, but doing so will not help improve our ability to get them well. Don't blame the lettuce. We have plenty of room for improvement in how we educate our patients.

12.1 "Dove or Ivory" versus "Dove, Not Ivory"

Patients teach us so many lessons. One of the more basic ones came from the mother of a child with atopic dermatitis. Her daughter's atopic dermatitis was flaring. She had already seen another dermatologist for treatment. The child's skin was very dry all over. We asked the mother what soap she had been using to bathe her child; she reported Ivory soap. We then asked her whether her prior dermatologist had recommended Ivory soap. "Yes," she said, "he told me to use Dove or Ivory."

That sounded odd. Common dermatology practice suggests using a less irritating soap such as Dove rather than one perceived as harsh and drying like Ivory. Would a dermatologist instruct a patient with atopic dermatitis to use "Dove or Ivory?" Unlikely. Instead, they had almost certainly suggested "Dove, not Ivory."

This example underscores the value of written instructions. If patients can misinterpret even the simplest instructions—if they can confuse "Dove, not Ivory" with "Dove or Ivory"—imagine how much more confused they must be when we state, for example, "Apply the Dovonex (calcipotriene) and the Ultravate (halobetasol) ointments twice a day, such as before work and before bed. Use them for about

DOI: 10.1201/9781003367628-15

two weeks or until most of the psoriatic plaques have been cleared. Then use the Dovonex twice a day on weekdays and the Ultravate twice a day on weekends. After some time, see if you can get by with the Dovonex alone." Can we expect patients to remember all these instructions, much less follow them?

12.2 Written Instructions

Do not leave adherence to chance. If our instructions are not in writing, all bets are off regarding what our patients will remember. When prescribing expensive biologic medications, we may tell patients, "Keep the medication refrigerated; do not freeze it." They may get home and wonder, "The doctor said something about refrigeration and freezing. Was it 'Do not freeze?' But why would they have mentioned it if I was not supposed to do it? And if refrigeration is good, freezing must be better." If we want our patients to remember information, we must put it in writing. We cannot expect them to remember what we tell them, especially in the stressful environment of a clinic visit.

Our interactions with patients suffer from the "curse of knowledge." This term refers to the psychological phenomenon in which people who know something cannot accurately imagine what it is like not to know. To us, proper use of medications is so ingrained that it is difficult, if not impossible, for us to imagine how foreign those concepts appear to patients. We must do more than just telling patients what to do. Patients hearing new information in the stressful setting of seeing a physician will often forget or, perhaps worse, misremember what they were told. Critical instructions should be provided in writing.

Distributing written instructions is easy for specialists who focus on a specific disease or perform a single procedure routinely. Mohs surgeons are particularly good at this. Much like McDonald's, Mohs surgeons do the same thing repeatedly. They can give their patients detailed pre- and post-operative instructions that are fully optimized and leave no doubts about what patients can expect and what they should do. General dermatology, though, involves a wide variety of diseases and medications, which makes it more difficult for us to give each patient personalized written instructions. While the task may be challenging, it is not impossible. With the implementation of electronic medical records, we can now even use smartphrases or templates to construct clearly written, standardized instructions for the wide variety of issues we manage.

12.2.1 Tear-Off Pads

One dermatologist suggested using a tear-off sheet of paper to transcribe information for patients. "The pads are in each room," she elaborates. "I started using them at the recommendation of my mother when I opened my practice. I had asked my mother what physicians have done for her that she found helpful over the years, and she said that our family pediatrician used these sorts of pads when I was a kid, and she found it enormously reassuring to have all instructions written down. I have had patients who have kept my instructions over the years to use as a reminder. One patient brought in psoriasis recommendations that I had made back in 1989 that he has kept in his wallet all these years!"

12.2.2 Sticky Notes

Another dermatologist employs a similar approach. "When I see an acne patient, I usually write down their regimen, on a sticky note if possible, so they can put it on the mirror in the bathroom." Besides, placing instructions on the bathroom mirror can serve as a convenient reminder for patients to use their medication. If we pre-print our office name and phone number on the sticky note, we can also do some marketing at the same time.

12.2.3 Avoid Writing "Use as Directed"

"Never write 'use as directed' on any prescription," suggested another dermatologist. "The half-life of their memory of how to use each topical medication is measured in minutes—hours, maybe. And the tube often ends up in a drawer full of other 'use as directed' tubes. Have a medical assistant both verbally explain and provide written directions for unique treatments such as soaks and bleach baths."

12.2.4 Digital Resources

Our modern world offers many informative digital and printed resources. The American Academy of Dermatology produces easy-to-read brochures. For patients with psoriasis, educational brochures from the National Psoriasis Foundation may be helpful (**Figure 12.1**). We can purchase print copies for our clinics or simply direct patients to the foundation's website (www.psoriasis.org).

Another digital resource, Vivacare (www.vivacare.com), offers a complete online library that can provide patients with personalized health information about their diagnosis and the recommended treatment plan (**Figure 12.2**). Alternatively, we can even create our own online resources for patients. The late Dr. Bill Danby of Manchester, New Hampshire, developed his own website (www.acnemilk.com) for educating patients about the causes of acne.

Electronic resources are evolving rapidly. Patients may already be able to ask ChatGPT what their diagnosis is and what treatment would be good and get answers that are surprisingly reasonable.

12.2.5 Pre-Printed Educational Materials

Pre-printed educational materials can be obtained from the American Academy of Dermatology, or we can prepare our own printed instructions.

Dr. Robert Brodell, formerly of Warren, Ohio, and later Chair of Dermatology and Pathology at the University of Mississippi, maintained drawers filled with educational materials in each of his examination rooms. Ensuring that the drawers were organized in the same fashion in each room helped him save time retrieving them (**Figure 12.3**).

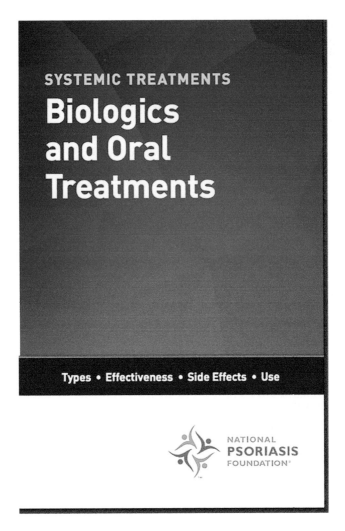

FIGURE 12.1 **The National Psoriasis Foundation brochure on systemic medications.** The foundation offers a wealth of educational materials including peer-reviewed brochures and fact sheets. We can hand out these brochures to inform patients about the benefits and risks of their medication as well as alternative treatments. (Courtesy of National Psoriasis Foundation.)

12.2.6 Written Action Plans

The treatment of asthma is complex and involves different medications for mainte-nance, mild flares, and severe exacerbations. Written action plans represent a pow-erful tool in treating children with asthma. They encourage parents to evaluate their child's breathing regularly using a spirometer and then to administer specific medications based on the spirometry readings. By outlining clear instructions, written action plans enable parents to administer the proper asthma medication in each scenario.

Your Information Prescription
Dermatology

The website below offers helpful resources about your health

______________________.vivacare.com

Skin Conditions
- ❑ Acne
- ❑ Actinic Keratoses
- ❑ Aging Skin
- ❑ Atopic Dermatitis
- ❑ Contact Dermatitis
- ❑ Fungal Skin Infection
- ❑ Hair Loss
- ❑ Hives
- ❑ Melasma
- ❑ Psoriasis
- ❑ Rosacea
- ❑ Shingles
- ❑ Skin Cancer
- ❑ Warts

Treatments
- ❑ Biologics for Psoriasis
- ❑ Biologics for Atopic Dermatitis
- ❑ Botulinum Toxin
- ❑ Corticosteroid, Topical
- ❑ Dermal Filler
- ❑ Isotretinoin for Acne
- ❑ Mohs Surgery
- ❑ Phototherapy

Skin Care
- ❑ Moisturizers
- ❑ Skin Self-Exam
- ❑ Sunscreens

Other ______________________

FIGURE 12.2 **A "prescription" for educational material.** Vivacare.com offers an entire online library of educational materials for patients. (Used with permission of Vivacare.com.)

Treating atopic dermatitis presents similar difficulties. Various agents—moisturizers, low- and medium-potency topical steroids, and non-steroidal topical immunomodulators—are used in different situations, depending on the severity and distribution of the lesions. A written action plan for atopic dermatitis can guide parents in applying the most appropriate agent (**Figure 12.4**).

12.2.7 Tailoring the Plan

One limitation of preset written action plans is that such plans may seem generic and not specifically targeted to an individual patient's special needs. That may be because different patients, despite their unique individual needs,

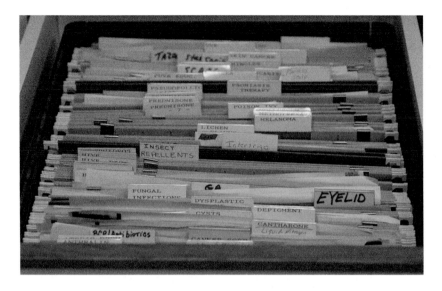

FIGURE 12.3 Pre-printed educational materials. Giving patients printed materials is much easier for a Mohs surgeon than for a general dermatologist who manages hundreds of diseases. While challenging, the task is not impossible. Organizing the drawers in the same way in each room can save time.

may need the same plan. For example, the great majority of patients with atopic dermatitis may need a moisturizer, some topical triamcinolone, and the use of mild cleansers. But patients may not be fully satisfied with receiving a generic plan.

One potential solution is to have several choices listed on the written action plan and just circle the same choices each time (**Figure 12.5**). Thus, the same standard plan is used for everyone, but patients aren't left feeling like the plan wasn't designed for specifically for them.

One study tested how satisfied people were with a standard treatment plan for atopic dermatitis compared to the same plan that was presented in the form of options circled from among several different choices (Bashyam and Cuellar-Barboza, 2020). The "placebo tailoring" improved both satisfaction with and confidence in the treatment plan.

12.3 Other Tools

12.3.1 Samples

Samples represent an excellent resource that we can utilize to teach our patients how to use their medication. They also facilitate adherence by circumventing the common problem of patients neglecting to fill their prescriptions.

Your Child's Eczema Action Plan

What is eczema?

Eczema, also called atopic dermatitis, is a chronic disease of the skin—meaning it is an ongoing problem. It causes dry, itchy, irritated skin and can be stressful for kids and families. **It is not contagious.** It sometimes runs in families, but not everyone in the family will have eczema.

Even though there is no cure, there are lots of good ways to control eczema. The BEST thing you can do for eczema is to keep skin moisturized! Kids with eczema have dry skin, and the drier the skin, the more itchy and irritated the skin will be.

Other instructions from your doctor:

_____
_____
_____
_____
_____

Here are some tips:

- Bathe daily. Use lukewarm water, 10 minutes or less.
- Use a small amount of mild soap. Choose one that is fragrance free. A liquid or bar is fine. Some that are specially made to be milder include: *Dove, Cetaphil, Purpose, Cerave*
- Pat skin dry—don't rub. Be gentle; rough rubbing can irritate skin.
- Moisturize. This is best done right after bathing, when the skin is still a little wet. Moisturize as needed throughout the rest of the day.
- Choose a moisturizer without fragrance. Here are some examples: *Eucerin cream, Cetaphil cream, Cerave cream, Aquaphor ointment, Vaseline petroleum jelly ointment*
- Choose fragrance-free soaps, moisturizers, & laundry detergent. Don't use dryer sheets; they are too irritating.

What to do in a flare:

Despite good routine care, your child's eczema may still flare. The plan below will tell you what medicines to use to get the flare under control. **Don't forget—keep using good routine skin care even during a flare!**

What to use during a flare:

_____
_____
_____

USE THESE MEDICINES FOR:

_____

If your child is not better by then, is getting worse at any time, or shows signs of infection (fever, chills, pus, or crusting), call your doctor at _____.

CALL US at _____ on: M–T–W–TH–F

Let us know how your child is doing overall.

Next appointment:_____

1. NORMAL/DRY:
Normal skin, a little dry, not itching much if at all.

PLAN:
- Regular skin care routine

2. MILD: Itchy skin with light redness.

PLAN:
- Regular skin care routine, but moisturize a little extra
- TRIAMCINOLONE 0.1% OINTMENT: use once a day until the itching is gone (use sparingly on face & gentials if needed)

3. MODERATE: Bad itching that keeps you and/or your child awake at night or causes scratching that leaves marks.

PLAN:
- Regular skin care routine, but moisturize a little extra
- TRIAMCINOLONE 0.1% OINTMENT: use twice a day until the itching is gone (use sparingly on face & gentials if needed)

4. SEVERE: Skin that is PAINFUL, RED, CRUSTED, or has PUS. Your child may have a FEVER or CHILLS.

PLAN:
- CALL YOUR DOCTOR TO SCHEDULE AN APPOINTMENT! Your child may have an infection requiring antibiotics.

FIGURE 12.4 A modified written action plan for atopic dermatitis. Written action plans are commonly used in asthma to help patients use the proper medication. The treatment plan varies based on the peak airflow measured via spirometry. Similarly, in atopic dermatitis, the intensity of treatment varies according to the severity and distribution of the lesions. (From Ntuen E, Taylor SL, Kinney M, et al., Physicians' perceptions of an eczema action plan for atopic dermatitis. *J Dermatol Treat.* 2010;21:28–33. With permission.)

12.3.2 Demonstrations

Some treatments, such as new biologic medications, require patients to perform tasks with which they are not usually familiar. Many patients have no experience

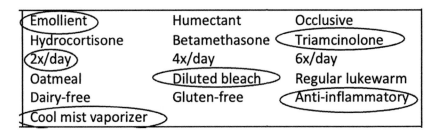

FIGURE 12.5 Placebo tailoring. By quickly circling the standard plan items, you can give patients the standard plan as well as a sense that this plan was chosen specifically to meet their individual needs. In addition, by having 4× and 6×/day options, the 2×/day option seems less cumbersome than it might if presented in isolation, as described in Chapter 14 on anchoring. A diet is included in the plan, as many patients desire dietary guidance, even though there is little evidence that any particular diet is helpful.

with self-injectable medications. One common practice is to show patients how to administer injections using a sample injector and some target object, such as an orange or grapefruit. The injector is placed against the orange, and the button is pressed. We wait until we hear the click, then we can dispose of the injector. Voila! The patient has been taught how to use the medication.

We should not educate our patients this way. Doing so leaves open the possibility that, on the way home, they will stop at the grocery store to purchase some citrus fruit. When they obtain their medication, they may inject it into the fruit and eat the fruit, thinking that was what we had instructed them to do (this happens!).

One patient reported that each time they used their self-administered biologic for their psoriasis, the administration was very painful, and the needle bent. That's right; the needle bent with each injection. (And this was not Bruce Willis's character in the movie *Unbreakable*, nor was it Marvel's Luke Cage.) The patient had been told to inject the medication in uninvolved skin, and the only uninvolved skin was on the top of the patient's head!

To avoid such misuse of the medication, it may be prudent to have a nurse administer the patient's first injection in the office. Then arrange for the patient to self-administer the next injection under nurse supervision. After that, hopefully, we can trust patients to do the administration properly themselves at home.

12.3.3 Teach-Back Method

Before we conclude the visit, we can ensure that our patients understand our instructions by applying the teach-back method. This method requires patients to express what they have understood and how they plan to use their medications while also inviting them to ask any questions. The technique is based on observations that students remember more when required to teach others about a topic they recently learned.

12.4 Cynical or "Pre-Educated" Patients

Some patients may not take their medication because they do not trust our knowledge of their medical condition. We can reassure these patients by showing them images of the condition from the web. Seeing one image on the web is often more convincing to a patient than all the explanation and reassurance that a physician can provide. Countless times, when patients have been unsure of whether the doctor had the diagnosis correct, patients have said, "Yes, that's it, all right! That's what I've got," after being shown one photo on the web. The web may have an "authority" with some patients that goes far beyond the authority of the human physician.

RECOMMENDED QUOTE

When patients proudly tell us that they have read WebMD before coming to see us, we should praise them: "What a relief! Finally, someone I can talk to at my own level! You would not believe how many patients come here without first taking time to educate themselves about their condition."

Other patients may have already educated themselves extensively before coming to see us and believe they know as much or more than we do about their problem. Our natural inclination might be to tell these patients how much training we have had, how much experience we have, how we know what the condition is and what needs to be done for it, and that they should trust us. Acting on those inclinations is a recipe for escalating conflict. A more effective approach might be to bite our tongues about our own knowledge and experience and instead praise our patients: "What a relief! Finally, someone I can talk to at my own level! You would not believe how many patients come here without first taking time to educate themselves about their condition." When we acknowledge and praise their knowledge, patients often will be far more receptive to our recommendations.

13

Helping Patients Remember

13.1 Like Us, Patients Are Forgetful

Many times, poor adherence is simply due to patients forgetting to take their medications. This obstacle is common yet understandable, given that we often recommend complex regimens that patients may find difficult to follow given their already hectic lives. In many instances, patients may not be in their optimal state of health to remember to take their medications regularly. Furthermore, we are creatures of habit. We go about many of our daily activities without even thinking about them. Starting a new medication is hardly automatic. Until taking medication is built into our routine, it will be routine to miss doses.

It may be beneficial to help our patients develop strategies to remember to take their medications. Unfortunately, there is no single technique or algorithm to identify which type of reminder may work best for a particular patient.

13.2 Using the Ikea Effect

We can apply the Ikea effect to help our patients remember to use the medications we prescribe. More specifically, we can ask them to come up with options to help them remember to take their medications; even if none of the options work particularly well, the process will promote a sense of involvement. It is important that we elicit these strategies from the patient, rather than imposing these on them. For example, instead of ordering patients to take their medication at the same time each day, we can politely ask them, "At what time of day did you decide to take the medication?" Another strategy might be to ask, "What method do you think would be best to help yourself remember to take your medication: a pill box, an electronic reminder, a sticky note, or a reminder from a family member?" The Ikea effect results in patients feeling more involved as they develop their own memory aids, and being more involved will make them more likely to adhere to treatment.

RECOMMENDED QUOTE

We should let our patients take the lead in developing reminder systems by asking, "At what time of day did you decide to take the medication?" or

DOI: 10.1201/9781003367628-16

"What method do you think would be best to help yourself remember to take your medication: a pill box, an electronic reminder, a sticky note, or a reminder from a family member?"

13.3 Tying Treatment to an Ongoing Behavior: Triggers

Getting patients to adopt a new behavior is daunting. Getting them to do something along with an existing behavior may be much easier. We can be creative. Simple memory aids and reminders are inexpensive ways to improve adherence. Such aids are commonplace in several spheres of daily living. Tying the treatment to a daily habit may be profoundly effective. Several potential approaches include the following:

1. Put acne medications by the toothbrush to help teenagers remember to use them twice daily.
2. Put a topical antifungal medication under the pillow to remember to apply it nightly.
3. After taking a morning medication dose, put the evening dose in your pocket. At night, empty your pockets before changing into pajamas and take the medications that remain.
4. Put the morning medication in or next to the clean, empty coffee pot. Take the medication before filling the coffee pot with water in the morning.

One dermatologist told us how her grandfather handled medication adherence: "Those pill sorters may help but can be difficult to open and may themselves present a barrier to adherence. My grandfather used to put all his medications for the day in a shot glass that he would leave on his kitchen table. At each mealtime, he would obtain the pills he was supposed to take. Whatever was left in the shot glass he would 'chug' at dinner. Yes, it is not the schedule his doctor envisioned, but Grandpa lived to be almost 100 years old." Another option is to tell people to duct tape the pills or topical medication to their toothpaste.

Many approaches can work. Triggers are very powerful tools, ensuring that patients do not move on to the next step of their daily routine without going through the medication. One of the authors of this book (Dr. Feldman) developed athlete's foot from doing Tae Kwon Do with his son. The condition required regular use of topical terbinafine to prevent recurrences. Remembering to use the medication was difficult, as Dr. Feldman would only notice the medication after putting his shoes and socks on (and was too lazy to take them off once they were on). Only after putting the medication on top of his socks in the sock drawer would he remember to use it faithfully. Putting the medication in the direct path of life can help patients use it better.

13.4 Packaging

What would drug packaging look like if we were trying to discourage patients from taking their medications? We would put medications in bottles of a bland color that blends in with the environment, easy to misplace and overlook, with caps that are difficult to remove. This description sounds a lot like our current medication bottles. It almost seems as though our current pill bottles were created with the goal of deterring patients from taking their medication regularly.

Perhaps more creative packaging designs can promote adherence by helping patients remember the proper dosing of their medications. Consider birth control pill packaging. When birth control pills were first approved, they came in bottles, and failure was common. Birth control pills are now very effective because of a change in packaging that results in excellent adherence. Because the pills are packaged in containers indicating which pills are to be taken on which days, adherence is quite good. The containers let patients know whether or not they have taken that day's dose. Similarly, the packaging design for initiating Otezla (apremilast) helps maximize adherence to a titration dosing schedule (**Figure 13.1**). This packaging is designed with three strengths of tablets arranged in the pattern the patient should follow for correct dosing to titrate up to the daily recommended therapeutic dose. Perhaps all oral medications should be packaged similarly.

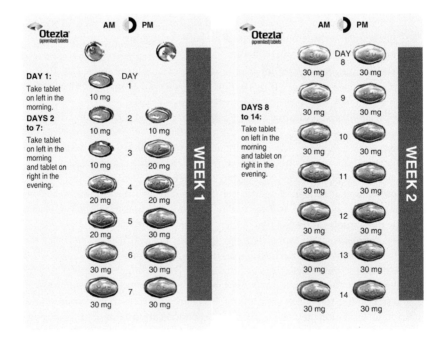

FIGURE 13.1 The Otezla (apremilast) initiation pack. This packaging is cleverly designed with three strengths of tablets arranged in a logical pattern based on the time of day, day, and week. Can you imagine how poor adherence would be if patients needed to remember this schedule and were just given the pills in a bottle? (Used with permission of Amgen Inc.)

Packaging medication in medicine bottles is asking for failure. Not only do the bottles not help patients remember to take medication, they also do not help patients remember if they took medication. Dr. Feldman is on a statin. He transfers his statin from the medication bottle sent by the pharmacy to a seven-day pill box to help assure that he takes the medicine. It is a huge help. If he sees that day's medication in the box, he knows to take it. If he doesn't see that day's medication in the box, he knows he already took it. Without repackaging the medication in the seven-day pill box, Dr. Feldman would miss doses and, possibly worse, would not remember if he took a dose even minutes after taking it, leaving him open to retaking the medication (possibly multiple times in one day) and overdosing.

13.5 Devices

A variety of devices may serve as helpful reminders for patients to use their medication. Many innovative products are available at www.forgettingthepill.com. Sensal Health is developing devices to help measure and improve use of topical treatments (**Figure 13.2**). These novel devices record when and how much medication is used, as well as giving patients reminders and feedback on their use of treatment (https://www.sensalhealth.com/post/learn-about-sensal-health).

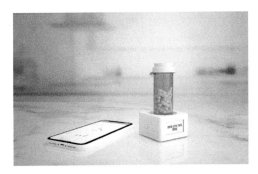

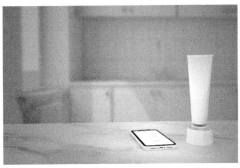

FIGURE 13.2 **Sensal medication monitors**. Sensal Health's electronic monitoring devices record the time medication is taken and the number of pills or amount of topical medication used (based on changes in weight). The Sensal devices also have visual and auditory alerts to remind people when medication is due to be taken.

Section 4

Psychology—Behavioral Techniques

DOI: 10.1201/9781003367628-17

14

Anchoring

The human brain isn't designed to assess absolute values; we assess things relatively. Despite being dramatically better off than cave-dwelling humans were 10,000 years ago, we're probably no happier now than we were then. We reset our baseline and judge things relative to that baseline. The human tendency to make relative—not absolute—judgments is critically important to how our patients think. Psoriasis patients with relatively mild disease may be unhappy; psoriasis patients who had very severe disease and now have only moderate involvement after treatment may be ecstatic with the improvement. Understanding that we evaluate things on a relative basis gives us a powerful tool to affect patient thinking.

Anchoring is a term that describes our tendency to use one piece of information (the anchor) as a reference point for determining the value of other items (Davis and Feldman, 2014). Most choices and decisions we make are based on an anchor, which serves as a foundation for making sound decisions.

Anchoring represents a common phenomenon that can be used to influence people's decision-making. For example, imagine that we are looking to buy a new jacket. We find a nice one normally priced at $495 but today marked down to $95; we would surely buy it. But if we saw that same jacket and were told, "It normally costs $35, but today the price is $95," there is no way we would buy it. But it is the same jacket being sold and the same $95 price in both scenarios. Objectively, other arbitrary prices should not affect our decision; a computer would evaluate the quality of the jacket and the current price and decide accordingly. But the human brain does not view the world so objectively. It considers the anchor, even if someone set the anchor with a completely arbitrary number.

14.1 Prescribing Injectable Biologics

Biologics are very effective for dermatologic diseases such as psoriasis, atopic dermatitis, and hidradenitis suppurativa, but patients are often fearful of injections. When we offer a once-a-month biologic treatment to a patient who has never received an injectable biologic, the patient's brain will be comparing taking an injection to not taking one. This comparison can be a frightening hurdle for a biologic-naïve patient considering biologic therapy.

This fear of injection is inherently subjective and can be easily modified. An arbitrary anchor can be used to reset patients' expectations and help them overcome their fear of injections. Imagine a scenario in which we wanted to start a monthly administered biologic such as secukinumab. We might say, "Biologics are like insulin; they are given by injection. You know how patients with diabetes give themselves insulin injections two to four times a day, right? Well, this medication is not exactly like insulin—you only need to take it once a month" (Lewis and Cardwell, 2018). After being anchored on the two-to-four-times-per-day dosing regimen of insulin, the brain is no longer comparing taking a shot to not taking a shot. Instead, it compares taking the monthly injection to a twice-daily injection, and suddenly, the monthly injection appears like no hurdle at all—a veritable bargain in terms of the frequency of injections. Objectively, the number of injections does not change; subjectively, the patient's perception of that number changes dramatically.

RECOMMENDED QUOTE

We can use anchoring to reduce the fear associated with injectable biologics by deftly explaining, "Biologics are like insulin; they are given by injection. You are familiar with how patients with diabetes give themselves insulin injections twice a day, right? Well, this medication is not exactly like insulin— you only need to take it once a month."

In one study, patients with psoriasis who had never received an injectable biologic were randomized into two groups. The first was asked how willing they would be, on a 1-to-10 scale, to receive an injectable biologic for their psoriasis once per month. The intervention group was asked the same question but was first asked how willing they would be to receive an injection for psoriasis once per day. Participants anchored to a daily biologic were much more willing (median, 7.5) to start a monthly biologic than those not anchored (median, 2.0) to the daily biologic (**Figure 14.1**) (Oussedik, 2017).

The anchoring phenomenon is familiar in pain perception with biologics. Patients who used prefilled syringes in the past often complain of greater pain with an autoinjector. However, patients starting with an autoinjector who have never received the prefilled syringe rarely complain about pain.

By the way, after reading about anchoring, you will notice the next time you see a product "on sale" that you are being manipulated. Yet despite knowing that the arbitrary retail price is simply a manipulation designed to get you to buy something, you will not be able to control the effect on your buying decisions.

Anchoring is a powerful tool. In addition to making injections more palatable, anchoring can be used to make the application of topical therapy more palatable. If we ask a mother to apply topical triamcinolone to her child's eczema twice a day, she may think, "I have to chase that kid down twice a day? This is a nightmare!" Instead, we can tell the mom, "I want you to apply this medication to your child four times a day: before school, have the school nurse do it at school, do it after school, and then again at midnight. Mom will think, "I have to get the school nurse to do this? What a nightmare. I'll probably have to miss work and make an appointment

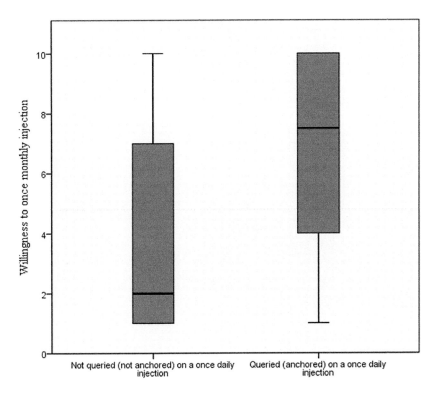

FIGURE 14.1 **Anchoring effect: Increased patient willingness to consider an injectable biologic.** Median willingness to a once-monthly injection in the control and intervention groups were 2.0 and 7.5, respectively; the distributions in the two groups differed significantly. Boxes indicate 25th and 75th percentiles; the horizontal line in the box indicates group median; the error bars indicate minimum and maximum values, excluding outliers.

to talk to the school nurse. There's probably a bunch of paperwork to do. I might have to get the paperwork notarized. I'm going to need a second container of medicine. This is a nightmare!" After giving Mom a few milliseconds to consider all that, we can say, "Wait, that's a lot. Let's just do it twice a day, once before school and then some time in the evening before bed." Mom will think, "Whew, that's better. I can do that easily." Anchoring can also be used to make medicines seem more effective or safer, just by presenting less effective or less safe options initially.

14.2 Ethics of Anchoring

After we diagnose a patient and offer the available treatment plans, the patient always has at least two options: accept or refuse therapy. Is it ethical for us to use psychological tools such as anchoring to "nudge" patients toward a particular treatment?

> A dermatology office had a sign
> in front of the entrance that read:
>
> ## Botox ®
> ## $249
>
> The practice obviously wanted to
> sell Botox.
>
> A more effective sign would have
> read:
>
> ## Botox ®
> ## ~~$499~~
> ## $249 special

FIGURE 14.2   **A Botox sale sign.** Using anchoring can make the price of Botox appear more appealing in a dermatology office.

Our utmost responsibility is to ensure that we provide our patients with optimal care. By utilizing anchoring deftly, we can guide patients into making the "right" decision regarding their health. There are always anchors. Patients will evaluate the options we present relative to any existing anchors. Our choice is not whether or not they will make judgments relative to an anchor, but rather whether to accept the existing anchor or to choose one that will best help the patient. If a particular anchor is more likely to lead to a better treatment outcome, it may be unethical not to use it.

As long as we are using these psychological tools purely for our patients' benefit, we are acting ethically. Would these tools help us sell more Botox (botulinum toxin)? Surely, they would (**Figure 14.2**). Would using them to sell more Botox be ethical? Now that is another subjective question. If you think using Botox helps patients improve their self-esteem and get the most out of life, you might think that helping the patient choose to receive Botox is an appropriate, ethical way to practice. If you are only prescribing Botox to help yourself put your children through college or pay for that second home, these approaches may not be appropriate. How we perceive these subjective issues is largely dependent on their context. (See Chapter 8: Setting the Right Office Visit Context for a reminder about the power of context in affecting our perceptions.)

15

Giving Salient Descriptions

Salience refers to the quality of standing out relative to other objects (Davis and Feldman, 2014). Our brains tend to hold on to ideas that create vivid picture in our minds. Human beings are more emotional than we are rational. The horrible news of a single beheading elicits a much stronger reaction than hearing about tens of thousands of lives lost from automobile accidents or heart disease.

15.1 Salient Adverse Effects

Our extensive training as medical professionals enables us to weigh the risks and benefits of treatment. Thus, it can be frustrating when we have the perfect treatment for a particular patient, only to hear them say, "No, I do not want to take that medication. I know someone who got cancer from taking that medication." The side effect may not even be related to the drug, and the person who experienced the side effect may be someone the patient met at a party or the grocery store. But with one salient event affecting the patient's perception, there may be no amount of data we could present that would change their mind. Since many of our new medications can be lifesaving and life changing, patients' tendency to turn down therapy can, in many cases, be downright painful for us as their caregivers.

Oral retinoids, such as isotretinoin, are used for the treatment of nodulocystic acne or acne refractory to other therapies. One publicized adverse effect from the use of isotretinoin is depression, and suicides, although rare, have been reported. Although the use of isotretinoin is closely monitored, the risk of serious depression is very low, and the drug likely prevents far more cases of depression than it causes, the salience of the isolated cases of reported suicides makes some patients reluctant to consider using the highly effective treatment.

The same might apply to the interleukin-17 receptor antagonist Siliq (brodalumab), a drug for psoriasis that was associated with four suicides in clinical trials (none of which were related to the drug in our opinion), resulting in a black-box warning about the risk of suicide. A black-box warning might terrify patients, despite the drug's benefits and the high likelihood that the suicides in the study were not caused by the medication. The black-box warning for suicide is not helpful; it might be better to have black-box warnings outlining the risks of not being treated or being undertreated, given the impact of psoriasis and its comorbidities.

Even when adverse effects are not as dramatic as suicidal ideation, they can be more salient than the benefits of the drug. The patient may have grown accustomed to suffering from the disease, and by comparison, the adverse effects may seem worse than the disease.

DOI: 10.1201/9781003367628-19

15.2 Using Salience to Our Advantage

15.2.1 Identifiable Victim Effect

The identifiable victim effect refers to our tendency to become moved more strongly by the experience of single identifiable victims than by statistics on large numbers of affected individuals. Consider the quote, "A single death is a tragedy; a million deaths are a statistic." Thinking about an identifiable victim moves us because it creates a vivid picture in our minds. Statistics, particularly large numbers, may provide greater scientific detail and information yet may be wholly unmoving to human emotion.

A salient, emotionally charged anecdote about an adverse effect stands out in patients' minds and is not easily overcome by reason or statistics. As a result, reciting data on the low probabilities of rare adverse effects can be a time-consuming exercise that is unlikely to change our patients' opinions. Instead of inundating our skeptical patients with data, we might respond with a salient anecdote or two of our own. We might point out an identifiable victim, such as a celebrity, who is doing well on the medication. Or we might state, "I had another patient a lot like you, and they had a rash very similar to yours and an excellent response to this medication. I think this medicine is a good choice for you." We might even add, "In fact, I think I saw that patient in this same examination room. Yes, they were sitting in the same chair you're sitting in now" to strengthen the perceived relationship (humans evolved as pack animals and have a strong tendency to perceive relationships to other humans on a very flimsy basis!). Salience is powerful, and it can work for us too.

RECOMMENDED QUOTE

If a patient fears a medication because a friend had a bad experience with it, it will be difficult to get the patient to consider that medication. One anecdote has huge effects on human thinking. We can use this phenomenon to our advantage, giving patients a salient anecdote of our own. We might say, "One of our other patients who reminds me of you and had a rash very similar to yours had an excellent response to the medication. In fact, I think I saw that patient in this same examination room."

The power of one anecdote to get patients to accept a new treatment should not be underestimated. The senior (that is, old) author of this book made a serious mistake trying to keep up with young people in a CrossFit class. The workout of the day was to do as many sets of five back squats and a 15-calorie row as possible in ten minutes. On the last back squat, something didn't feel right in his lower back. A few days later, while walking along the streets of Shanghai after sitting for 18 hours on the plane ride to China, footdrop set in. After the return flight and another 18 hours of sitting, during clinic, the disc found the nerve. Intense sciatica pain began. It was so intense that the author's staff had to wheel him around in a wheelchair to see patients. Leaving clinic early to go to the urgent care center, he demanded narcotics for the pain. Despite the narcotics, he couldn't sleep at night, so he read UpToDate on how to manage sciatica. He was hoping to read that he could have back surgery with no risk, no downtime, 100% chance of immediate pain relief, and full, permanent recovery. That's not what UpToDate offered. UpToDate said, "Do physical therapy." He read the references UpToDate cited. He did his own literature searches. Well-controlled clinical trials and a wealth of other data, which he read in excruciating detail, proved beyond a shadow of a doubt that, of the available medical, surgical, and therapy options, the best thing he could do was physical therapy. So he resigned himself to seeing a physical therapist.

Sometime later, back at work using a walker, he ran into his partner, the Mohs surgeon. The Mohs surgeon said he, too, had had a disc problem: it was in the neck; it had adversely affected his motor function; he had seen neurosurgeons who prescribed him prednisone; and with prednisone, he had gotten better right away.

Thus, the senior author of this book had, on the one hand, read all the evidence proving beyond a shadow of a doubt that he should do physical therapy and had, on the other hand, one anecdote from someone he had little to nothing in common with (the author is a medical dermatologist, and the Mohs surgeon is, well, a Mohs surgeon). What did our author do? Of course, he took the prednisone.

Telling patients one anecdote about a "similar patient" with a "similar rash" who did well with a particular treatment is more effective than data could ever be. This principle was tested in a study comparing how comfortable people would be with a therapy after hearing data versus an anecdote versus the anecdote plus the data (Johnson, 2021). Patients felt more comfortable with the treatment after hearing the anecdote than after hearing the data, whereas the anecdote plus the data was no better than the anecdote alone.

15.2.2 Encouraging Sunscreen Use

We can also put salience to use by changing how we encourage sun protection to prevent skin cancer. When motivating patients to wear wide-brimmed hats and apply sunscreen regularly, saying, "Use sunscreen so you do not get skin cancer" is often an exercise in futility. Instead, we might tell them, "Make sure you use sunscreen so you do not develop a golf ball–size, ulcerating, odious, pus-draining tumor on your nose, requiring a major surgery that would involve removing the whole nose, leaving a gaping, dark hole in the center of your face, but it is not so bad because the rubber prostheses they make these days look almost exactly like a normal nose!" While the statement, "Use sunscreen so that you do not get skin cancer" also covers this horrible outcome and many others, the more colorful, anecdotal description paints a picture in patients' minds that they will not easily forget.

RECOMMENDED QUOTE

Instead of simply telling patients to use sunscreen to prevent skin cancer, we can apply the principle of salience by telling our patients, "Make sure you use sunscreen so you do not develop a golf ball–size, ulcerating, odious, pus-draining tumor on your nose, requiring a major surgery that would involve removing the whole nose, leaving a gaping, dark hole in the center of your face!"

15.2.3 Reducing Tanning Bed Use

We can also use salience in developing public health cancer prevention strategies. The prospect of developing skin cancer, which usually occurs decades after using tanning beds, may not be salient enough for young tanning bed users. Young people may feel that the short-term benefit of a tan outweighs the long-term risks of skin cancer. However, physical appearance is highly salient, and educational programs that drive home the negative impact of ultraviolet exposure on skin beauty may be more salient and effective (Feldman, 2001). Moreover, presenting the effect of tanning as a loss of youthful appearance may be more powerful than explaining that giving up tanning is a great way to prevent skin cancer. We discuss the benefit of presenting information as losses rather than as gains in the next chapter.

16

Emphasizing Losses versus Gains

Loss aversion describes the human preference for avoiding a loss rather than obtaining a gain of comparable size (Davis and Feldman, 2014). This bias can lead to an irrational inconsistency as our preferences can shift drastically in response to small changes in the presentation of two mathematically identical propositions.

16.1 The Statin Scenario

For instance, imagine a scenario in which we wish to initiate a statin in a patient with hypercholesterolemia. We can expect that controlling the disease with a statin would improve a patient's lifespan by reducing the likelihood of a heart attack or stroke. Assume, hypothetically, that taking the statin would give the patient an expected lifespan of 81 years, whereas not taking it would yield a predicted lifespan of 79 years.

There are two distinct yet mathematically identical ways to present these numbers. We could explain, "If you take this statin, your cholesterol will improve, and you can expect to live two years longer." Alternatively, we could say, "If you do not take this statin, you can expect to die two years earlier." Although the two propositions are mathematically identical, we perceive them very differently. Living, on average, two years longer is a nice bonus—on the other hand, if we think of it as two years longer in a nursing home, it might not sound so good—but we absolutely don't want to die two years earlier.

16.2 Loss Aversion in Dermatology

16.2.1 Selecting an Appropriate Treatment

Loss aversion is most apparent in dermatology patients whose disease requires aggressive treatment yet who exhibit a bias toward accepting less treatment. Some patients remain extremely reluctant to use treatments associated with potential adverse effects, even if the treatment results in less suffering than the disease itself. It can be heartbreaking to witness a patient with severe psoriasis who chooses to continue suffering by opting for topical therapy instead of considering systemic therapy out of disproportionate fear of adverse effects.

One reason patients may refuse a therapy is that they evaluate treatment decisions as being between a benefit of the treatment (gain) and a side effect of treatment (a loss). It may be helpful to forge a dynamic in which the patient chooses

DOI: 10.1201/9781003367628-20

between two losses, as opposed to a gain and a loss. Rather than emphasizing the gain of improving the severity of the disease, we might counsel patients, "This drug can prevent your disease from growing even worse," or "If we don't use this drug to treat your condition, you will almost certainly continue to suffer from the disease; if we do use it, there is some risk of a side effect." Faced with the possibility that their disease may progress or cause continued suffering versus the rare risk of a side effect, patients may become more inclined to avoid the loss caused by the disease rather than avoiding the potential loss from an adverse event of the medication that isn't likely to occur.

16.2.2 Encouraging Medication Use

To encourage patients to use their medication, we can also frame the event as preventing a loss rather than resulting in a gain. In motivating a patient with psoriatic arthritis to take methotrexate, for example, we might avoid saying, "Take this pill so that you maintain joint function." Instead, we might explain, "Take this pill so you do not lose the function of your hands." Although there is no practical difference in the outcomes described by the two presentations, patients may perceive a substantial difference.

RECOMMENDED QUOTE

It may be more impactful to phrase outcomes of treatment as losses instead of gains. We can explain, "Take this pill so you do not lose the function of your hands," instead of "Take this pill so that you maintain joint function."

16.2.3 Focus on Short-Term, Not Long-Term Risks or Benefits

While loss aversion can aid in promoting sunscreen use and other preventive health behaviors, focusing on long-term risks (or benefits) may not be particularly impactful. For example, to encourage patients to use sunscreen and avoid tanning beds, we can emphasize the short-term threat of losing the youthful elegance of their skin. Citing the example of a celebrity who lost their youthful appearance prematurely due to sun damage might be even more persuasive. In contrast, describing how sun protection reduces the long-term risk of skin cancer may have little effect on patients, as events that may occur years later are heavily discounted in perceived importance.

Moreover, patients may discount the future much more than physicians do (Feldman, 2002), making behavioral changes that seem sensible to physicians for their long-term benefit seem completely irrational to patients. It should not be surprising that our admonitions to eat healthy, get regular exercise, use sun protection, and quit smoking based on the long-term benefits of such behavioral changes aren't particularly effective. We may be more effective in encouraging healthy behaviors if we can find short-term benefits of the recommended behaviors, such as having a better chance of getting a date this weekend.

17

Framing Risks of Side Effects

17.1 Probability Bias

We don't talk about it much here in North Carolina, but if you believe in evolution, you can imagine Cro-Magnon man counting mammoths going by. "One, uh, two, uh, three, uh, a lot!" Early man probably didn't count past ten and certainly had limited use for numbers like one hundred or one thousand. Humans did not evolve to use big numbers. Most humans probably had no use for such big numbers until very recently in our history. It shouldn't be surprising that we just aren't that good at putting data into perspective.

Modern life has increased the frequency of situations in which we encounter significantly large or extremely small numbers or probabilities, such as the US deficit stretching into the trillions or new medications conferring a 1-in-1,000 risk of an adverse effect. Our brains are not designed to grasp such large numbers or minuscule fractions. This explains why people play the lottery when there is only a 1-in-500,000,000 chance of winning a fortune. For all practical purposes, a 1-in-500,000,000 chance of winning is essentially zero. More people are struck by lightning . . . twice! But people think about the possibility of winning, imagine what it would be like to win, and the thoughts fill their cranial cavity like an expanding balloon, leading them to act as though there is some significant chance of winning.

Extreme numbers, large or small, lead to probability bias. Probability bias describes our response to situations in which we either magnify a small risk, defined as regressive bias, or mistakenly treat different-size risks as equal, known as probability neglect (Davis and Feldman, 2014).

17.2 Fear of Side Effects

Humans tend to overrate the importance of rare events, including rare side effects; this is a form of regressive bias. A particular medication's side effect may only occur in 1 patient out of 1,000, but people's minds tend to focus on that 1 rather than the other 999. The rare side effect may paralyze patients' willingness to take an otherwise very safe medication.

Since fear alters patients' perception of reality, our job is to calm their fears and give them a more realistic understanding. If patients are overly afraid of the risks of a particular treatment, we must change their perceptions of these risks if we hope to

DOI: 10.1201/9781003367628-21

get them to use their medication. Giving patients a clearer perspective of the risks can help them understand that these risks are well worth it when considering the potential benefits of therapy (and the high risk of not taking treatment).

17.3 Framing

Framing is our tendency to change how we value a set of options based on our current frame of reference or the frame from which the option is presented. Framing is a vital strategy to express small risks in terms that our patients can comprehend.

17.3.1 What "Sounds" Safer?

A patient once presented to our clinic with severe psoriasis needing biologic treatment. However, he would not consider taking any biologic. Ingrained in his mind was the possibility that biologics could cause liver disease, a side effect that he must have had conflated with that of methotrexate. We could not tell him there was no risk of liver disease (as anyone can get liver disease), so we asked him if he would take the medication if there were only a 1-in-1,000 risk of liver disease. Slamming his hand down on the table, he exclaimed, "No! You are not listening to me! I had a relative who died of cirrhosis. It was a slow, painful, lingering death. I would never take that chance!" We then asked him, "I understand. What if we had a different biologic with which 99 out of 100 do not get cirrhosis; would you take that?" "Sure," he replied, "I would take that."

What an odd but typically human way to view these numbers! A drug with which 99 out of 100 have no problem is ten times riskier than a drug that confers a 1-in-1,000 risk of an adverse event. Nevertheless, stating that "99 out of 100 do not have a problem with the drug" sounds safer than characterizing the risk as 1 out of 1,000. If we are told 99 out of 100 do not have a problem, we picture the 99. If we are told 1 in 1,000 does have a problem, we fixate on that 1, especially when it is a highly salient, rare outcome laden with emotional baggage.

17.4 Framing the Risks of Biologics

Patients may be terrified by rare adverse events associated with biologics, such as infection or malignancy. Accurately explaining the risks of biologics, or any other medication, is a challenge. However, even scarier than quantitative yet accurate descriptions of side effects are ambiguous ones. Vague descriptions may be magnified out of proportion, leading to disproportionate fear of our proposed treatment regimens. If patients hear, "There is a risk of lymphoma," they may behave as if there is a 50–50 risk. Warning patients about a "risk of lymphoma" may be a good way to discourage a patient who does not need a biologic from taking one, even if the biologic has no known risk of lymphoma—inflammatory diseases have a risk of lymphoma, so there is a risk of lymphoma, even if it does not come from the biologic.

Due to our inherent probability biases, it can be difficult for us to use numbers alone in describing the risks of treatments in ways that put those risks into an accurate perspective. For this reason, it is important to communicate the risks in other ways. Emphasizing that the risk of an adverse event is like a familiar event characterizes it more accurately: "The risk of lymphoma from taking the medication is comparable to that of having a fatal accident while driving on a highway." Visual materials can aid in illustrating the true size of miniscule fractions (**Figure 17.1**) (Kaminska, 2013).

17.4.1 The Patient Who Needs a Biologic

Imagine if a patient with severe psoriasis were to ask, "Biologics increase the risk of infection, right?" An appropriate and reassuring response might be "There is a potential risk of infection, but if you look at 100 people who use a biologic for a year, 99 of them do not get an infection." If we are trying to be even more reassuring, we might say, "Because you have so much psoriasis, your immune system is out of whack, and right now you have about a 1-in-100 chance of developing a serious infection. But if you take this all-natural, organic anti-inflammatory agent made from living cells, it will complement your natural healing mechanisms and rebalance your immune system, and 99 times out of 100, you will not get a serious infection."

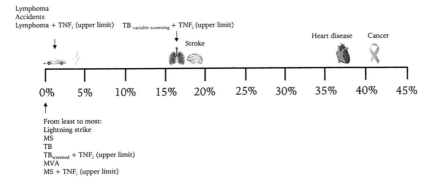

FIGURE 17.1 Using visual aids to clarify risks. This graph compares the lifetime risks of tumor necrosis factor (TNF) inhibitors in psoriasis patients to more common benchmarks of risk. Abbreviations: MS, multiple sclerosis; MVA, motor vehicle accidents; TB, tuberculosis; TNF$_i$, TNF inhibitors.

RECOMMENDED QUOTE

In reassuring patients about the risks of biologics, instead of explaining that there is a 1-in-100 chance of infection, we could state, "If you look at 100 people who use a biologic for a year, 99 of them do not get an infection."

If a patient shows a strong preference for no treatment at all to avoid a "risky" drug such as a biologic, we should emphasize that continuing to suffer with the disease is not a risk-free course of action either. Many dermatologic diseases increase the risk of comorbidities, and successful treatment of the disease greatly alleviates this risk. For example, psoriasis is an independent risk factor for the development of obesity, metabolic syndrome, cardiovascular disease, depression, and suicide. In these cases, successful treatment of patients' psoriasis, even with treatments that are not risk-free, might have some potential to reduce patients' overall risk of morbidity and mortality, although strong evidence of a risk reduction benefit is not yet proven.

17.5 Decoding Patients' Language

There are code words in dermatology that signify danger to our patients. One such word is *steroid*. We often use the term instead of the far more unwieldy word *glucocorticosteroid*. For mothers of children with atopic dermatitis, the seven letters of the word *steroid* may connote danger. Fear of steroids is common and a frequent cause of poor adherence (Brown and Rehmus, 2006). The word *steroid* may evoke visions of East German female Olympic swimmers with muscular physiques and hairy faces or of Barry Bonds and other steroid-abusing baseball players. No good comes from uttering the word *steroid* to a mother in describing a treatment for her child. Unless we are telling her about a medication that is "not a steroid," we should avoid using the term. We can sense how scary the word *steroid* is to mothers when, after we have prescribed triamcinolone to her child, she immediately asks with trepidation, "Is this a *steroid*? The last dermatologist wanted me to put a *steroid* on my baby."

When asked a question we do not want to answer, we can use an approach widely used in U.S. presidential debates and taught in media training classes: just answer a different question. We do not have to lie and say it is not a steroid. We can just let that question go by, gently put our hand on the mother's shoulder, look her in the eye, and reassure her, "It is a cortisone medication, sort of like over-the-counter hydrocortisone, only a little stronger." If she seems especially afraid, we might even explain, very gently, "This is an all-natural, organic, gluten-free, topical anti-inflammatory agent made in a nut-free facility designed to complement your child's natural healing mechanisms. It brings the immune system back into balance [while moving our arms like a see-saw moving into balance] and harmony [while clasping our hands at the chest/heart] because we like to take a holistic approach to the management of skin disease in children."

RECOMMENDED QUOTE

Instead of uttering the word *steroid* in front of a fearful mother, we should explain, "It is a cortisone medication, sort of like over-the-counter hydrocortisone, only a little stronger." For mothers who are particularly afraid, we can go even further: "This is an all-natural, organic, gluten-free, topical anti-inflammatory agent made in a peanut-free facility designed to complement your child's natural healing mechanisms and rebalance the immune system and bring it into harmony because we like to take a holistic approach to the management of skin disease in children." We would not lie and say, "No, it is not a steroid."

In asking about a "steroid," she is really asking, "Is this safe to put on my child?" When we answer, "It is a cortisone medication" or "It is an all-natural, organic, topical anti-inflammatory agent," we are telling her, "Yes, it is safe." We can go over the long-term side effects in more detail at the next visit, after she has seen how well the medication works in the interim.

17.6 Perceptions of Risks

Interestingly, the mere perception of a potential risk, even when no risk exists, can strongly influence patients' willingness to use a medication. For example, the information on the package inserts for the topical calcineurin inhibitors Protopic (tacrolimus) and Elidel (pimecrolimus) suggests that their use is associated with an increased risk of lymphoma.

Aside from animal data demonstrating lymphoma formation at a dose 47 times higher than the maximum recommended human dose, there is strong evidence that there is *no increased incidence* of lymphoma with topical tacrolimus or pimecrolimus (Siegfried and Jaworski, 2013). In post-marketing studies, the risk of cancer in patients treated with these medications was lower than in patients who did not receive these agents (Fleischer, 2006). Yet the perception of risk has reduced our inclination to prescribe these medications and patients' willingness to use them. Even the non-risk of lymphoma with topical tacrolimus and pimecrolimus remains terrifying!

18

Using Side Effects to Our Advantage

Patients can sometimes be terrified of medication side effects. If we tell a mother we are prescribing a "steroid" for her child, she will almost assuredly not apply the medication due to fear of side effects. She will not listen to anything else about the treatment—she will just think about "steroids." The medication is likely to stay in the container, assuming the prescription is even filled. Yet side effects are not all bad.

Although side effects can scare patients, they also represent a powerful tool. We can use jiujitsu on side effects, turning their power to stop people from using medicine to get people to use medication better. Side effects, we can tell patients, are positive signals that the medication is working.

18.1 Topical Agents That Sting

In some cultures, it is commonly believed that if we do not feel a sensation, nothing is happening. Perhaps for this reason, some shampoos are even marketed to cause "tingling." For patients who expect to feel a sensation, adding menthol to their topical agent may give them an immediate sense that the medication is working. The sensation created by the menthol may even have direct effects on pruritus.

Some medications prescribed in dermatology do sting without the addition of menthol, particularly alcohol-based solutions applied to broken skin. More specifically, the alcohol-based products prescribed for scalp psoriasis can sting considerably, at least initially. Dr. Richard Fried, of Yardley, Pennsylvania, suggests warning patients, "This medication is so strong it may sting when you first start using it."

Since so many patients are afraid of strong steroids, I prefer to tell patients, "The stinging is a sign the medication is working," which is true because the stinging is a sign the patient successfully applied the medication to the scalp, where it is working. Too often, the medication ends up on the hair where it doesn't do anything. When that happens, there is no stinging. Stinging is a sign the medication is working.

There's another way to use side effects with us macho men who would "tough it out" to avoid admitting weakness. We can often turn this maladaptive behavior on its head by challenging them, "This cream may sting. Many men do not have what it takes to use it. Do you think you can do it?"

We can take the challenge of a side effect and turn it into an opportunity to improve the patient's adherence to treatment. Whenever there is an expected side

 DOI: 10.1201/9781003367628-22

effect, it may help to let patients know up front: "You may experience side effect X. In my experience, it is a sign the medication is working." For our scalp psoriasis patients, we can say, "This medication may sting, but that is a sign the medication is working." While this statement is a bit of a stretch, it is nevertheless true—if the medication is causing stinging, the patient is applying it correctly to the scalp (not just to the hair), and if the medication is getting onto the scalp and into the skin, then it surely is working.

RECOMMENDED QUOTE

For patients with scalp psoriasis who are using alcohol-based products, we can use side effects to advantage by stating, "This medication may sting. It is a sign the medication is working."

18.2 Other Side Effects

Some acne therapies, such as oral isotretinoin, may cause dryness. Whether this dryness actually helps improve the acne remains uncertain, but if the patient believes it is associated with improvement, it may encourage them to continue using the medication. Topical 5-fluorouracil, used to treat actinic keratoses, is one of the most irritating medications we prescribe, yet adherence to it is surprisingly good (Yentzer and Alikhan, 2009). It may be that the irritation serves to remind people to use the medication. Letting them know that "the irritation is a sign the medication is working" may further encourage good use of the treatment and a willingness to put up with the side effect.

Topical minocycline can cause the skin to have a yellow color. Not warning patients about this may lead to treatment discontinuation when the effect occurs unexpectedly. Warning patients of the potential side effect in advance may help. Framing the side effect as an advantage may be even better: "This medication is a yellow acne mask designed to give good acne control."

A dermatologist in Dallas, Texas, suggested a most innovative use of an adverse effect to improve patient adherence. When prescribing spironolactone to treat acne in women, we can inform them, "Unfortunately, this drug is also a diuretic. In addition to its effect on your acne, you may notice some weight loss." This statement serves as an excellent example of using an adverse effect to promote adherence. A similar statement could be made when discussing Otezla (apremilast) for the treatment of psoriasis, as taking apremilast can also be associated with weight loss. More commonly, apremilast is associated with nausea and headaches. We can let patients know that, in our experience, these side effects are a promising sign that the drug is working.

The effect of describing an adverse event as a signal of efficacy was tested in a survey of adults with self-reported atopic dermatitis (Bashyam and Cuellar-Barboza, 2020). Subjects reported their willingness to use a topical treatment on a scale of one (strongly not willing) to nine (strongly willing). If the cream did not cause a painful sensation or caused a non-painful cooling sensation, mean reported willingness to use the cream was about seven on the nine-point scale. If the cream caused discomfort and the patient was not warned in advance, willingness to use it was only about four. If the cream caused discomfort and the patient was warned in advance, willingness to use it was only about five. But if the cream caused discomfort and the patient was told in advance that the discomfort was a sign the medication was working, willingness to use it was seven. Jiujitsu! Letting the patient know the stinging was a sign the medication was working alleviated its negative effect on willingness to use the medication (at least, it did in the survey).

Section 5

Special Considerations

DOI: 10.1201/9781003367628-23

19

Patients with Psychiatric Conditions

Psychological factors frequently occur in patients with dermatologic disease and can influence patient adherence. Consequently, we must routinely screen our patients for psychosocial issues that may affect adherence and attempt to understand how these issues can make adherence difficult for them.

19.1 Depression

Depression exacerbates psoriasis. Some dermatologists believe depression affects psoriasis through "psychoneuroimmunologic" mechanisms, pointing to evidence that antidepressants can improve psoriasis. More likely, depression worsens psoriasis by reducing adherence. Patients with depression are less likely to muster the energy or motivation to use their medications. In these patients, antidepressants may improve psoriasis indirectly by improving patients' ability to use their medication.

19.2 Stress

Stress commonly exacerbates psoriasis. Psychoneuroimmunologic mechanisms may be at work here as well, but poor adherence provides a simpler explanation for the effect of stress on psoriasis. Under increased stress, patients are less likely to remember to take their medication, and thus, adherence worsens.

19.3 Personality Disorders

19.3.1 Obsessive-Compulsive Personality Disorder

Patients with obsessive-compulsive personality disorder are a dream in terms of adherence. They exhibit rigid conformity to rules and procedures, perfectionism, and excessive orderliness. These patients likely floss their teeth every day. We can rest assured they will use their medication.

Patients with an inclination toward an obsessive-compulsive personality are fairly easy to identify. They often work as accountants, engineers, architects, and

DOI: 10.1201/9781003367628-24

maybe pilots too. During their visit, they may even show us a spreadsheet, meticulously created on Microsoft Excel, listing every medication they have ever tried and categorized using multiple colors.

Not only can we count on obsessive-compulsive patients to use their medication, but we can also enlist their help in ensuring that others take their medication. Some of our most adherent patients have a spouse with obsessive-compulsive tendencies. For patients who have proven unreliable, we can make their obsessive-compulsive spouse responsible for ensuring they use their medication.

19.3.2 Antisocial Personality Disorder

Patients with antisocial personality disorder lie at the opposite end of the personality spectrum. Antisocial personality disorder is characterized by a disregard for social rules, societal norms, and cultural codes as well as impulsive behavior and indifference toward the rights and feelings of others. Patients with this personality disorder will not use their medication and will feel comfortable lying to us about it. These patients need a short adherence leash. We should give them easy-to-use, fast-acting medications. If they fail to respond quickly, it may be best for us to resort to office-administered treatments.

19.4 Delusions of Parasitosis

One of the most challenging conditions to treat in dermatology is delusions of parasitosis, or Morgellon's disease (Feldman, 2016). In this nightmare of a disease, patients describe experiencing the sensation of organisms crawling on their skin, which can cause severe picking and insomnia.

Anti-psychotics may prove useful in treating delusions of parasitosis. However, prescribing these medications can be difficult because patients are often reluctant to accept treatments that contradict their disease model as they believe the disease is caused by parasites rather than the mind. Accordingly, when discussing anti-psychotics, we could explain, "The parasites seem to be irritating the nerves in your skin and are causing you a lot of itching. We should try a medication to calm down these nerves." We can even explain, "Pesticides are used to kill bugs. Most pesticides work by targeting the nervous system, so we will need to use a medication that works on the nervous system of whatever bugs or worms are there. We cannot use regular insecticides because they are poisonous to humans too. But we can use medications that work on the nervous system. While these drugs are normally used in psychiatry, we can use them in you to get rid of the bugs." Because patients with delusions of parasitosis usually exhibit poor insight, we wonder if long-acting depot anti-psychotics might be a reasonable option in these patients to maximize adherence and give them the best treatment outcomes.

RECOMMENDED QUOTE

We can broach the topic of starting an anti-psychotic by saying, "Pesticides are used to kill bugs. Most pesticides work by targeting the nervous system, so we will need to use a medication that works on the nervous system of whatever bugs or worms are there. We cannot use regular insecticides because they are poisonous to humans too. But we can use medications that work on the nervous system. While these drugs are normally used in psychiatry, we can use them in you to get rid of the bugs."

20

Pediatric Patients

Adherence in pediatric patients is particularly complex. For one thing, we are now working with two distinct audiences—the child and the parents. Even more, these parties may not cooperate with each other.

As children grow older, they increasingly assume responsibility for adherence. In younger children, problems with adherence usually originate from parents' difficulties in administering the medication, and it may be helpful for us to ask parents about their struggles or proactively provide strategies that avoid potential hurdles. For older children, the problem more often arises from the child rather than from the parent. For example, an adolescent might report having taken medications when, in fact, they had not. We must recognize a growing child's role in adherence and address issues pertaining to both the child and the parents.

20.1 Young Children

20.1.1 Assigning Parental Responsibility

Medication use in young children is totally dependent on the parents. Pediatric oncology research on adherence to chemotherapy for leukemia show that adherence can be worse in two-parent households than in single-parent households (Bhatia, 2014). What could explain this finding? In single-parent households, it is clear who is responsible for adherence. In two-parent households, each parent thinks the other is in charge, so there is a diffusion of responsibility. Each parent may think the other will give the child the medication, resulting in no medication being given; alternatively, each parent may feel responsible for giving the medication, and medications may be given twice! Therefore, when we are treating children who come from two-parent households, we might ask which parent will be primarily responsible for adherence.

20.1.2 Empowering Young Children

One mother, a physician, shared her own story about the treatment of her son's atopic dermatitis:

> I am a full-time anesthesiologist with administrative duties. My son was 12 at the time, a good kid and generally responsible for himself. My son manages his asthma with two medications daily without prompting. He asked to see someone for the dry, itchy skin he had on the inner folds of his elbows. These had turned white and thickened.

Looks like eczema, I thought, and I made an appointment to see our dermatologist, who is my good friend. We saw the dermatologist, got a prescription for triamcinolone ointment, got it filled, handed it to my son, and I am thinking my job is done. Not a crazy thing to do, given that he manages his asthma with two medications and a rescue inhaler with little input from me.

One month later, we go for our follow-up visit, and his elbows look pretty much the same. He stated that he had lost his triamcinolone three weeks ago while on a cruise with his grandparents and that he did not tell me because he thought I would become irritated. This situation was personally embarrassing as a mother and a physician to stand in front of my colleague and friend in medicine with my non-compliant son. "How can you possibly expect the eczema to improve if you do not even use the medication? Why are we even here if you lost your medication? This is a waste of everyone's time," I voiced.

I think my dermatologist had seen this movie before. "You do not have to use the triamcinolone," the dermatologist told my son. "Your eczema is not contagious, and it will not kill you. If it really bothers you, have your mom get the medication again and use it when you need it. If it does not bother you, leave it alone. It is really up to you."

Six months have gone by, and my son's eczema is still gone. He uses the triamcinolone on his own schedule. I think it was helpful for him to feel empowered about whether he uses it.

20.2 Praise and Self-Monitoring

Praise is cheap, and it can be a strong motivator. Whether we are with our patients or our office staff, we should freely give recognition for good work. Similarly, when patients are improving, we should congratulate them for using their medication correctly.

Praise is particularly valuable in treating conditions in children. They crave recognition and are driven by even the smallest bits of positive reinforcement. Once children are old enough to be involved in their own care, we can administer praise by giving them awards as part of a self-monitoring program.

20.2.1 Sticker Charts

The power of sticker charts as motivators should not be underestimated. If we were to propose using sticker charts in a research study, the human subjects research committee might reject the study on the grounds that sticker charts are overly coercive.

When caring for young children, a sticker chart may be just what we need to get them to take their pill or apply their topical medication. It can be as simple as drawing a one-week calendar grid with squares for each day of the week (two squares each day for a twice-daily medication) or using a calendar. We can provide

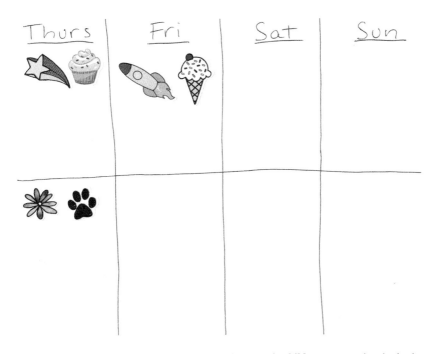

FIGURE 20.1   A sticker system for improving adherence in children. A pre-printed calendar or hastily drawn grid, along with some age- and gender-appropriate stickers, are all that parents need. Few things motivate children as much as the recognition they feel when they receive a sticker rewarding them for their good behavior.

some stickers, say some blue Teenage Mutant Ninja Turtles stickers and some pink *Frozen* stickers (we leave the choice of the stickers to the child and, being woke, don't make any *a priori* gender-based assumptions about which ones they would prefer). We can have the parent give the child a sticker each time they use the medication, up to twice a day (**Figure 20.1**) (Luersen, 2012).

Sticker charts give children a sense of pride and accomplishment while also encouraging continued adherence. Behaviorally speaking, they positively reinforce adherence by pairing a reward with the desired behavior. Moreover, the resulting chart may provide a somewhat reliable record of how well the medication is being used. Developing a sticker chart routine with patients takes merely a few minutes that might otherwise be spent adjusting medication regimens that provide little benefit. Children with atopic dermatitis are a good target population for this intervention, which affords them autonomy and allows them to relish the recognition of their accomplishments.

20.2.2 Packaging

If we were to design the ideal packaging of triamcinolone for use in young girls with atopic dermatitis, the medication might come in a bright pink container with a medication bottle cap that, when opened, plays music from the movie *Frozen* (sadly, the most effective packaging idea we could come up with for boys would be a pistol-shaped applicator that shoots the medicine onto the skin, and we don't want to promote that). Such packaging might make children much more excited about using their medication. The industrial-looking white jars that are typically used seem unlikely to generate any enthusiasm. Surely, we can do better.

While unit-dose packaging of topical treatment may not be practical, such packaging would likely have a large effect on adherence. Seeing which dose should be taken at which time on which day could be a useful and effective motivator and reminder for better adherence and outcomes.

20.3 The Rebellious Teenager with Acne

Teenagers are in a transition period between the dependency of childhood and the independence of adulthood. They have a desire to assert their independence. They are also overly concerned about fitting in with their peers. Hormones are raging as part of puberty. These hormones not only make them moody and brittle but also cause acne. Of all the places where the acne could appear, it primarily inhabits the face, the area of the body that affects how we perceive ourselves, how others perceive us, and, most importantly, how we perceive others perceive us.

As if this coalescence of factors was not enough, the lesions on the teenager's face may be more distressing to the parent than the child. The mother may feel the lesions need to be cleared to assuage her feelings of guilt about the condition. Moreover, her child is transforming into an adult, and sometimes she does not want to accept this reality. She may not be ready to give up control. The interaction between a teenager attempting to achieve independence and a controlling parent can end in loud confrontations.

Imagine a teenage boy, sitting on the end of the examination table with a baseball cap pulled down low over his face. Long and bushy hair protrudes from underneath the cap. With the shadow cast by cap and the long hair, his face is shrouded in darkness, making evaluation of the acne nearly impossible. His mother is sitting on the other side of the room with an angry look on her face. "Tell him to use the medication," she says in an irate, forceful tone. "He is not using it the way you told him!"

He doesn't wear the cap to hide the acne; nor is his hair long to hide the acne. He wears a hat indoors because it bothers her; moreover, if she is a New York Yankees fan, it's usually a Mets hat. His hair is so long because she demands he cut it short. Of course, he is not using the medication. He is not using the medication because his mom is telling him to use it. At every opportunity, the child is attempting to assert independence, even if it means suffering with more acne.

20.3.1 Improving Adherence in Adolescents

No controlled studies have been performed to assess interventions for poor adherence associated with a controlling mother, but logic dictates asking her to distance herself from the situation. Doing so allows us to assign responsibility to the adolescent, making him accountable for whether the acne improves and whether to use the medications or not.

In her review on improving adherence to acne treatment, Dr. Hilary Baldwin offers several suggestions to improve adherence in teenagers with acne (Baldwin, 2006):

1. Maximize the quality of the office visit, focusing attention on the patient-physician relationship.
2. Recognize self-conscious patients' need for modesty.
3. Give patients control over their care.
4. Involve patients in the choice of vehicles.
5. Make patients better as soon as possible so that they see that the medication works.
6. Do not waste time pushing ineffective treatments.
7. Recognize patients who do not want to be treated.
8. Educate patients thoroughly and carefully, dealing with anticipated side effects proactively.
9. Confront non-adherence.
10. Examine non-adherent behavior.
11. Create a contract with patients.

While teenagers are highly resistant to overtly strong messages telling them what to do, they desperately seek the acceptance of their peers. For this reason, normative behavior may be a valuable tool. We can advise teenagers, "This medication will give you control over your acne the way other kids have control. It is the medication most other teenagers use in this situation." We would NEVER tell them, "Most teenagers are not getting better because most of them are not using their medications." Teenagers want to be like other teenagers.

RECOMMENDED QUOTE

Because teenagers love to fit in with their peers, we can tell them, "This medication will give you control over your acne the way other kids have control. It is the medication most other teenagers use in this situation."

One study examined techniques to improve adherence in teenagers with acne (Yentzer and Wood, 2011). The group of teenagers whose parents received daily phone calls telling the parent, "Do not forget! Remind your child to use the medication," had significantly worse rates of adherence than the group of teenagers who received no daily reminders. A similar study found that daily text message reminders are ineffective in improving adherence to topical acne medications. Perhaps teenagers perceive the daily reminders as irritating, triggering a sense of resistance and thereby reducing adherence. Conversely, a weekly web survey designed to hold teenagers accountable doubled adherence (**Figure 20.2**) (Yentzer and Wood, 2011).

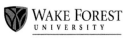

Acne Survey

SCHOOL *of* MEDICINE
DIVISION *of* PUBLIC HEALTH SCIENCES

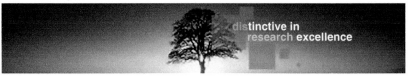

Thank-you for participating in our web survey!

Please select the answers that best apply to your experience with the medication this week, and click submit.

1. How many days did you apply the drug this week?

2. How easy was it to use the study drug as prescribed?

3. Did using the medication interfere with your daily routine?

4. How useful wat the medication in treating your acne?

5. How severe is your acne now?

6. Have you had any side effects?

   If yes, what side effects did you experience?

submit

FIGURE 20.2 Use of a web-based survey to improve treatment outcomes for teenagers with acne. A web survey can make teenagers more accountable for the use of their medications. Patients who were sent the survey asking them to report their progress exhibited two times higher adherence than those not sent the survey.

Teenagers, like all patients, need reminders, but they do not like being told what to do. So, rather than suggesting that they use a reminder system, we might say to them, "Most teenagers find it helps to have a reminder system. Some put the medication next to their toothbrush, others put a sticky note reminder on their mirror, and others put the medication on their pillow. I do not know which method would work best for you. When you come up with one that works well for you, would you please send me a text message to tell me about it? Your approach might help some of my other patients."

21

Suddenly Adherent Patients

While improved adherence typically leads to better treatment outcomes, suddenly improved adherence in previously non-adherent patients can have unanticipated, serious adverse effects due to excessive drug exposure.

21.1 "Resistant" Hypertension

When patients reduce the use of their medication without informing us, we may increase the prescribed dose of the medication or prescribe additional medications to help control the condition. For example, consider patients who appear to have resistant hypertension, defined as having a blood pressure above goal despite at least three optimally dosed anti-hypertensive medications of different classes. We may prescribe multiple agents at high doses to control the hypertension.

However, the reason their blood pressure is "resistant" to treatment may be poor adherence. When such a patient is admitted to the hospital for some other medical condition—for example, pneumonia—the intern or hospitalist might write orders to give the patient all the outpatient anti-hypertensive drugs they had been prescribed, and the patient may take all these anti-hypertensive medications together for the very first time. This sudden increase in adherence may cause severe hypotension that sends the patient to the intensive care unit.

21.2 Epilepsy Camps

Similar sudden increases in adherence can occur in children with chronic diseases who are sent to a medical camp. For example, consider children with epilepsy who are poorly adherent to their anti-epileptic regimen and thus have breakthrough seizures. Because these children take their medications before the office visit, blood levels of their seizure medicine taken at the visit are invariably in the therapeutic range. The physician concludes the drug isn't working, and additional treatment is needed. To control the breakthrough seizures, a second or third anti-seizure drug may be prescribed but remains rarely taken.

Then, when these children attend a summer camp for kids with epilepsy, they may develop toxic drug-blood levels. Being at camp may be the first time these kids regularly take the prescribed doses of all their anti-epileptic medications. Encountering children with lethargy and other signs of medication overdose is common in this setting.

DOI: 10.1201/9781003367628-26

22

The Most Adherence-Resistant Patients

Some patients are extremely resistant to using their medication. They may be very forgetful. They may be very leery of medication side effects. Others may simply not want to get better due to secondary gain. Nevertheless, we can use certain approaches to assure good adherence in even the most adherence-resistant patients.

22.1 Hospitalization

For some patients, the best option may be to relieve them of their responsibility for taking their medications. Self-administered treatments can be substituted with physician-administered treatments. For example, when topical therapy is not working for a localized inflammatory process, the agent is likely not being applied. It is for this reason that atopic dermatitis rapidly improves when the patient receives topical triamcinolone in the hospital. In this case, hospitalization is a very effective, albeit expensive, way to ensure adherence—the medication is applied regularly by the nurses. Home health services may be appropriate for some patients and offer similar benefits.

22.2 Office-Administered Treatments

Hospitalization or home health services, though, are typically not necessary. Indeed, in many cases, the patient can simply come to the office to have the treatment applied.

22.2.1 Topical Therapy

For patients with localized psoriasis "resistant" to topical steroids because of poor adherence, we might recommend phototherapy and have our nurse apply the topical agent before each phototherapy session. We could explain to our patients that applying the medication helps the ultraviolet light penetrate the skin more effectively. In clinics without standard phototherapy equipment, we could even apply the topical agent in the office and use a handheld light device, such as a Wood's lamp, to deliver the "phototherapy" treatment. In this scenario, the light itself may be irrelevant; when the patient comes to the clinic, it gives us a chance to apply the topical agent. The plaques will then exhibit very rapid improvement, even when the same topical therapies were ineffective when prescribed for self-administered use.

DOI: 10.1201/9781003367628-27

22.2.2 Methotrexate

If a patient is receiving methotrexate for psoriasis, lichen planus, or another inflammatory disease, and the medication is not working as expected, do not assume the disease is resistant to the medication; the patient might simply not be taking it. It is hard to blame patients for being terrified of taking their methotrexate at home after we tell them about the potential risks, such as cirrhosis, pancytopenia, and pulmonary fibrosis.

An alternative is to switch the methotrexate from oral administration to weekly intramuscular injection. However, be sure to watch out for adverse effects. If the patient has "failed" 15 mg/week of oral methotrexate because they were not using it, a dose of 15 mg/week of intramuscular methotrexate may be too high. In other words, consider reducing the dose when switching from patient-administered to physician-administered treatment. In a previously non-adherent patient, new-onset optimal adherence can have serious consequences. Refer to the previous chapter, Chapter 21: Suddenly Adherent Patients, for more on this topic.

22.2.3 Biologics

When self-administered biologics are seemingly losing their effectiveness in a particular patient, consider the possibility of poor adherence. Changing to a new treatment or complicating the regimen by adding treatments may not be necessary.

Patients with severe psoriasis may benefit from the TNF inhibitor Remicade (infliximab), which is administered intravenously at infusion centers, or the interleukin-23 antagonist Ilumya (tildrakizumab), a subcutaneous injection that is only approved for administration by a healthcare provider. However, patients can develop resistance to infliximab for reasons other than poor adherence, such as the formation of anti-infliximab antibodies. For these patients, it may be helpful to add methotrexate in combination with infliximab to reduce the likelihood of developing resistance. If the patient is at high risk for poor adherence, methotrexate can be given intramuscularly in the office too.

RECOMMENDED QUOTE

We can broach the topic of administering self-injectable medications in the office by explaining, "Sometimes when patients administer the medication themselves in the home, it does not always get to the part of the skin where it works best. For the next few weeks, our nurse will give you the injection."

Other TNF inhibitors, such as Enbrel (etanercept), Humira (adalimumab), and other newer biologics for psoriasis are not associated with the same degree of antibody-mediated treatment resistance seen with infliximab. Nevertheless, the efficacy of these agents may also decrease over time, possibly due to antibodies but also possibly due to poor adherence to drug administration or poor handling of the drug. Patients may put the drug in the freezer, or, even if they refrigerate the drug, the refrigerator temperature may be set too low—we've all seen bottles of water in our refrigerator freeze if kept too close to the coils.

Although etanercept and adalimumab are normally patient-administered medications, it may be reasonable to have a nurse administer the medication in the office. We might explain to our patients, "Sometimes when patients administer the medication themselves in the home, it does not always get to the part of the skin where it works best. For the next few weeks, our nurse will give you the injection." Another biologic, Stelara (ustekinumab), is commonly given as an office-administered injection; better adherence to ustekinumab could be one explanation for the better persistence to ustekinumab treatment when compared with persistence to anti-TNF drugs used for psoriasis (Sandoval, 2013).

Section 6

Illustrative Cases

DOI: 10.1201/9781003367628-28

23

Pediatric Atopic Dermatitis

Atopic dermatitis is very responsive to mid-potency topical steroids such as triamcinolone. Even severe atopic dermatitis rapidly clears with inpatient application of topical steroids. However, many patients have a disease "resistant" to triamcinolone prescribed for outpatient use. Such resistance can oftentimes be attributed to poor adherence, but patients and their caregivers often remain adamant that the steroid was ineffective, assuring us that they used it correctly.

Poor adherence in atopic dermatitis may be due to a wide array of factors—complex instructions, lack of trust in us, displeasure with the topical agent vehicle, steroid phobia, and cost of the medication. Nevertheless, simple measures may promote adherence.

23.1 Case Description

A two-year-old girl came to clinic accompanied by her foster mother reporting a two-year history of unremitting, unrelenting eczema, mostly affecting the extremities but also involving the trunk (Lewis and Feldman, 2018). The mother, a registered nurse, reported that the lesions had persisted despite applying triamcinolone 0.1% ointment twice daily for nearly two years. Skin examination revealed typical eczematous lesions on the extremities in an extensor distribution (and no striae, which might have been expected had triamcinolone been used twice daily for nearly two years). Her disease was particularly severe around the ankles, with overlying crust and excoriations.

The mother, quite convincingly, insisted that the triamcinolone ointment had been ineffective. When asked who had been applying it, she reported she had been applying it personally on her daughter's skin. She was queried for missed doses, but she insisted that she had been applying it twice daily. When asked how much of the medication she had purchased, she described obtaining the recommended amount.

Given her report that the topical triamcinolone had failed, we instructed the mother to apply clobetasol 0.05% ointment twice daily, report how it was working after three days, and subsequently return to applying triamcinolone following the brief course of clobetasol.

The next day, the mother sent us an email message, reporting, "You were absolutely right about the triamcinolone ointment! We were previously told to only use it 'sparingly.' . . . I think I just was not using enough of it for two years. . . . Her eczema looks so much better even after 24 hours! . . . I will not be filling the prescription for clobetasol. Clearly you were right, and all she needed was a more liberal application of the triamcinolone. I am so glad we came to see you yesterday!"

DOI: 10.1201/9781003367628-29

23.2 Case Reflection

23.2.1 Shortening the Treatment Time Horizon

Suggesting that our patients apply a topical agent for six to eight weeks, as is often recommended for atopic dermatitis, would place a large perceived treatment burden on the patient or caregiver. On the other hand, encouraging communication within three days of the visit shortens the treatment time horizon. It alleviates the psychological burden associated with long-term adherence while also fostering accountability during the early stages of treatment. It also enables the patient to witness the rapid benefits of well-used treatment and become assured that this treatment is effective when needed. Perhaps the mother had envisioned the frightening prospect of having to apply a seemingly dangerous "steroid" to her daughter's youthful skin for years. Shortening the treatment time horizon, though, allowed her to focus on the more feasible task of applying the ointment for a mere three days without fear of long-term side effects. As a result, the infant's lesions resolved in a single day after reportedly persisting for nearly two years.

23.2.2 Simplifying the Treatment Regimen

It is also important to avoid complicating the therapeutic regimen. Adding moisturizers, complicated bathing regimens, humidifiers, specialized clothing, wet wraps, topical calcineurin inhibitors, penetration enhancers, or more potent topical steroids only makes adherence more difficult. Successful treatment simply involves getting the patient or parent to apply the mid-potency (or low-potency for infants) topical steroid. The most practical approach is to limit treatment to a single steroid to be used once or twice a day for a few days. By eliminating all ancillary medications and emollients from the regimen, the parents can direct their attention entirely to using the topical steroid, after which the atopic dermatitis may clear beautifully in a few days.

23.2.3 Legitimizing the Concerns of the Parents

While it is important to simplify the treatment regimen, it is equally important to legitimize the parents' concerns. In our case, recommending clobetasol served as a way of affirming that we listened to the mother's report of her experience with the triamcinolone. If we had simply suggested continuing to apply triamcinolone, even after her insistence that it had not been working, she would likely perceive us as insensitive to her concerns. Adherence is markedly lower in atopic dermatitis when mothers perceive that we did not consider their input in designing treatment plans (Fenerty, 2013). Since parents are intimately involved in treatment, we must adequately address their concerns if we wish to maximize adherence.

23.2.4 Establishing A "Blame-Free" Environment

One component of a strong doctor–patient relationship involves creating a "blame-free" environment. We must broach the topic of adherence without shaming or accusing patients. In one study, the only circumstance in which questions about adherence were not perceived negatively was if a "de-shaming" communication style was used (Barfod, 2006). Assigning culpability for treatment failure is destructive to our relationship with our patients. It engenders feelings of guilt and forces patients to become defensive, reducing the likelihood that they will adhere to our treatment plan. A more effective strategy is to praise parents for being proactive and concerned about their child's health. Such praise builds trust and strengthens the physician–patient relationship.

24

Skin Cap for Psoriasis

24.1 Exciting News of Skin Cap

In March 1997, Drs. Dorinda and Walter Shelley wrote in their diary published in *Cutis*,

> The big news is Skin Cap, coming out of Spain, now sweeping the country as an over-the-counter spray therapy for psoriasis. Make no mistake about it; it is good. One of our friends said, "I don't have any psoriasis practice. They all use Skin Cap." . . . No longer do the patients need steroids inuncted, ingested or injected, and no more methotrexate or PUVA visits. It seems unbelievable that a product not even requiring prescription can be so effective.
>
> (Shelley, 1997)

The product was a zinc pyrithione spray that also contained the detergent sodium laurel sulfate. When the Shelleys gave it to a patient for large psoriatic plaques on the legs, the plaques virtually disappeared after one month of using a one-second spray twice a day. They reported on another patient with scalp psoriasis:

> Last week one of our patients jumped up when we entered the room to exclaim, "It's a miracle," as she showed us the spray can. Her psoriasis of the scalp, which had been modestly improved under our treatment for several months, was now gone. It had taken just four days.

Skin Cap showed unprecedented efficacy. In a study demonstrating its histologic effects on psoriasis (Rowlands, 2000), Dr. Bill Danby observed histologic improvement in as little as five hours. Within two weeks, nearly all the histologic features of psoriasis had completely resolved. Skin Cap was a revelation for dermatologists, improving psoriasis that had been resistant to all other previous treatments.

Then came the shocking news that the product contained clobetasol propionate (Smith, 1997; Swanson, 2005). To many dermatologists, this news did not make sense. They had been prescribing clobetasol propionate in the form of ointments. The new spray therapy somehow appeared to be more potent than the clobetasol ointment ever was. Given the impression that moisturizing ointments are more potent for psoriasis than drying sprays, there had to be something else that had made the product so effective.

DOI: 10.1201/9781003367628-30

24.2 Why Was Skin Cap So Effective?

Some dermatologists thought that it was perhaps due to a higher concentration or greater bioavailability of clobetasol in the Skin Cap preparation, but studies comparing the delivery of clobetasol with Skin Cap to that of branded clobetasol preparations revealed no greater penetration with Skin Cap (Franz, 2003). Others believed that perhaps the zinc in Skin Cap exhibited a synergistic effect with the clobetasol, an interesting hypothesis given the presence of "zinc fingers" in corticosteroid receptors. One study tested this hypothesis in patients with bilaterally symmetric psoriasis lesions (Housman, 2003). Lesions on both sides of the body were treated with clobetasol foam; one side also received a spray of zinc pyrithione, and the other side was administered vehicle spray. The side treated with zinc did marginally *worse* than the side not treated with zinc; there was no sign the zinc augmented the effect of topical clobetasol.

What could explain the unparalleled efficacy of Skin Cap? There were likely three reasons why Skin Cap exhibited greater efficacy than the prescribed topical clobetasol products.

First, better adherence. The spray formulation of Skin Cap was easy to use. Although we are often taught to prescribe ointments for psoriasis, many patients are reluctant to apply ointments, given their greasy nature. The spray was easier to apply and far less messy; thus, patients were more likely to use it.

Second, better adherence. Patients likely used Skin Cap regularly because they were less fearful of its adverse effects. When prescribing clobetasol ointment, we often tell patients, "This ointment is the most powerful steroid known to humans. If you use this for more than two weeks, seriously bad things are going to happen to you." These warnings are reinforced by the package insert, which shows even more ominous side effects. Consequently, patients likely did not apply the ointment regularly and returned to the office claiming, "I used the medicine, but it did not work. We need to try something else." With Skin Cap, we essentially told patients, "This spray cannot hurt you. It contains the same active ingredient as Head & Shoulders shampoo." Patients used it regularly, and their psoriasis rapidly improved.

Third, you guessed it, better adherence. Patients likely applied Skin Cap frequently because they had paid for it themselves. When patients purchase a medication, they are more likely to use it. A similar phenomenon occurs during physician dinner lectures and continuing medical education events. When doctors are not charged a fee when registering in advance, they are less likely to attend the event than if a registration fee, however small, had been charged.

When people are invested in something (even if it is a tiny investment), it has a big effect on their behavior. Some years ago, the Wake Forest Dermatology Department held a psoriasis treatment continuing medical education (CME) meeting on a Saturday in January. We had a lot of external financial support and didn't want to charge attendees a fee. Our CME office said we needed to charge a fee; if we didn't charge a fee, they said, we ran the risk of no one showing up. So, we charged a $15 fee for the six hours of CME credit. There was a freak ice storm that weekend, yet the meeting was still well attended. Despite the ice, one dermatologist from West Virginia came, at the peril of his life, over the ice-covered mountain roads to attend the meeting. It's nearly certain he would have stayed at home if he hadn't had $15 invested in attending.

24.3 Lessons from Skin Cap

The effectiveness of Skin Cap illustrates that psoriasis, even its most resistant types, can be cleared quickly when patients use a potent topical anti-inflammatory treatment regularly. This finding has been amply demonstrated in research studies with non-moisturizing clobetasol preparations. In these studies, clobetasol spray and foam products are very effective. In trials investigating the efficacy of two different forms of clobetasol—Olux foam and Clobex spray—psoriatic plaques are clear or almost clear in 60–80% of patients in two to four weeks (Feldman, 2007; Reid, 2005; Beutner, 2006; Warino, 2006). That's faster clearing than with our fastest-acting biologic treatments.

A very large community trial revealed that 80% of plaques cleared or almost cleared with four weeks of using twice-daily clobetasol spray (Lebwohl and Colon, 2007). This high degree of efficacy was observed in newly diagnosed patients in addition to patients who were previously treated with and resistant to other topical therapies, phototherapy, or systemic therapies; 80% clear or almost clear in one month is more effective than our most effective biologics! More recently, a trial studying twice-daily topical desoximetasone spray showed that it alone can clear or almost clear psoriatic plaques in nearly 40% of patients in four weeks (Saleem and Negus, 2018).

The efficacy of topical clobetasol when applied as prescribed should not be surprising. Imagine if oral prednisone 1 mg/kg/day were administered for psoriasis. While systemic steroids are not used in psoriasis due to potential adverse effects, the psoriatic lesions would probably clear very quickly. Assuming 100% absorption, no first-pass hepatic metabolism, and uniform drug distribution, the tissue concentration in the skin from a 1 mg/kg dose should be roughly 1 mg/kg or 10^{-6} g per gram of tissue. In contrast, the concentration of topical clobetasol is 0.05%, or 5×10^{-4} g/gm—500 times higher than the 1 mg/kg with oral prednisone—not to mention that clobetasol is many times more potent than prednisone at activating corticosteroid receptors. Although clobetasol is not fully absorbed, it is applied directly to diseased skin, which exhibits an abnormal barrier function that facilitates penetration. Accordingly, topical clobetasol should be extraordinarily effective for localized plaque psoriasis. And it is, but only if patients apply it.

Topical clobetasol does not need to be prescribed as an ointment. A topical agent does not necessarily have to moisturize the plaques; after all, methotrexate or biologics can clear psoriasis without moisturizing the lesions. The patient simply needs to apply the clobetasol to areas of diseased skin. If a patient prefers an ointment, then we should prescribe an ointment. But Skin Cap teaches us that if patients do not want to use an ointment, then a less messy clobetasol product may represent a more effective treatment option.

25

Coral Reef Psoriasis

Psoriatic plaques sometimes have the morphology of a coral reef with very thick adherent scale—so-called coral reef, ostraceous, or rupioid psoriasis. One dermatologist said that coral reef psoriasis is a sign of resistance to topical therapy because the medication just can't penetrate the thick scale. That dermatologist was, we believe, half right. This kind of psoriasis is a marker for resistance to topical treatment but not because of poor penetration. Diseased skin, even with this thick scale, has poor barrier function. The medication probably would penetrate just fine if medication were applied. But patients who let their plaques get this thick are probably not applying the treatment. Coral reef psoriasis is a sign of resistant disease because it is a sign the patient may be non-adherent to treatment.

25.1 Case Description

A 42-year-old male presented with very thick, scaly psoriatic plaques, primarily affecting the knees (**Figure 25.1**) (Feldman, 2008). He had failed multiple topical agents. Treatment with Enbrel (etanercept) 50 mg twice weekly produced mild, temporary improvement. Oral prednisone had been added briefly but also failed to control the lesions. Several treatment options—oral retinoids, phototherapy, and a variety of topical agents and vehicles—were discussed.

In lieu of prescribing phototherapy or a systemic agent, we gave sample bottles of a non-messy, clobetasol propionate 0.05% spray, instructing him simply to apply it, and nothing else, twice daily. We did not prescribe a descaling agent. Giving a descaling agent would have complicated the treatment, and this patient already had the coral reef sign of resistance to treatment. We wanted to keep the treatment simple. We scheduled a return visit in three days, expecting that the short time to the return would encourage excellent use of the treatment.

When he returned, the lesions showed marked improvement, with further improvement after two weeks of use. The patient reported that he had used the spray as directed by itself, finding it much more appealing and practical than the messy ointments that had been prescribed in the past.

25.2 Case Reflection

The presence of coral reef–like lesions served as a tip-off that his psoriasis had been resistant to treatment because of poor adherence. Patients who allow their

DOI: 10.1201/9781003367628-31

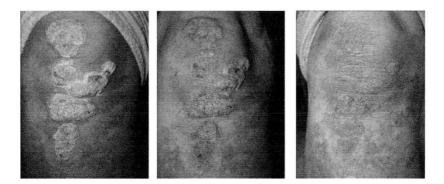

FIGURE 25.1   Treatment of "coral reef" psoriasis with clobetasol propionate 0.05% spray.
Plaques with rock-like, coral reef scale (left-most image). At three days, the lesions showed marked improvement with clobetasol propionate spray twice daily (middle image). After two weeks of continued treatment, the lesions exhibited considerably more improvement (right-most image). (From Feldman SR, Brown KL, Heald P. "Coral reef" psoriasis: a marker of resistance to topical treatment. *J Dermatolog Treat.* 2008;19(5):257–8. Reprinted by permission.)

plaques to grow this thick are clearly not using their medication. The poor barrier function of even thick psoriatic lesions readily permits penetration of topical steroids, if the medication is actually applied. For these patients, we need to start by making sure they trust us. Then we must find a vehicle they will use well, such as a non-messy topical steroid. Finally, we should schedule an early return visit to establish accountability for early adherence.

Moisturizers and descaling agents may offer some benefits in dry, scaly conditions, but they are not necessary for the management of inflammatory conditions. If we were to assume that the lesions were resistant to treatment because of poor penetration, we might devise a complicated regimen involving anti-inflammatory and keratolytic agents. Complicating the treatment regimen, though, reduces adherence, yielding worse outcomes than a simpler regimen. A single topical steroid, without keratolytics or an ointment vehicle, may be sufficient. In our patient, recommending a spray as opposed to an ointment made it easier for him to use the steroid. Giving him the medication directly obviated the problem that he might not fill the prescription. Lastly, suggesting that he return in three days shortened the treatment time horizon. After experiencing rapid improvement, his confidence in the medication increased; thus, he continued to use it. He had an excellent outcome, despite being "resistant" to so many other therapies in the past.

At an international meeting of dermatologists, there was a forum on management of scalp psoriasis. A top expert from Italy said that to treat scalp psoriasis, treatment must start with urea, a keratolytic, to remove the thick scale that prevents medication from penetrating. A top expert from France agreed, though he recommended topical salicylic acid, not urea. Another expert, from French-speaking Canada, one who does many clinical trials, said he agreed with the French dermatology expert. Dr. Feldman, one of the authors of this book, retorted, "That's crazy. That just makes the treatment more complicated. I just recommend the topical clobetasol and get the patient to use it." The Canadian dermatologist said in response, "But if you don't remove the scale, the medicine won't penetrate." Dr. Feldman replied, "You are famous for all the clinical trials you do." "Yes," responded the Canadian. "And you've done many studies of topical steroids for scalp psoriasis," Dr. Feldman said. "Yes, that's true," the Canadian responded. "And in those studies, you just give the topical steroid alone, without any penetration enhancer, because the protocols don't allow concomitant therapy," Dr. Feldman said. And the Canadian dermatologist responded, "Yes, that's right. And the patients improve quickly in those trials. You must be right. Patients don't need the penetration enhancer."

For "treatment-resistant" diseases like coral reef psoriasis and scalp psoriasis, the resistance is often due to poor adherence to treatment. We discuss scalp psoriasis treatment, the mother of all compliance problems, in more detail in the next chapter.

26

Scalp Psoriasis

Of all the conditions in dermatology, scalp psoriasis is one of the most frustrating disorders, for patients and dermatologists alike. Dr. Feldman began to subspecialize in psoriasis in the early 1990s. While treatment seemed to improve most forms of psoriasis, it always seemed as if scalp psoriasis never got better. Nothing left Dr. Feldman feeling more inadequate as a dermatologist than taking care of patients whose scalp psoriasis could not be controlled. Holding conversations with other dermatologists and attending American Academy of Dermatology meetings provided no answers. None of the treatments *en vogue* had worked, including oral anti-fungal agents, keratolytics, topical steroids in all sorts of vehicles, Dovonex (calcipotriene) solution, and all sorts of drug combinations including "triple gel therapy"—a mixture of Lidex (fluocinonide) gel, Keralyt (salicylic acid) gel, and Estar (coal tar) gel. For twelve years, the cure for scalp psoriasis had been elusive, and Dr. Feldman suffered under a cloud of inadequacy, seeing dozens of patients with scalp psoriasis who were simply not improving despite all his efforts, including very complicated treatment regimens where he would throw the whole kitchen sink at the problem.

Then the answer suddenly seemed apparent. Dr. Feldman had been invited to present a lecture on scalp psoriasis for patients at a national meeting organized by the National Psoriasis Foundation. The venue was a large room lined with rows and rows of patients with scalp psoriasis. Standing at the podium, He began, "Scalp psoriasis is so frustrating." This introduction was meant to show the audience that they were listening to a caring, empathetic doctor. The entire room of heads nodded in agreement. "It is not just frustrating for patients, but it is also frustrating for us dermatologists, too. We like to see our patients get well, and scalp psoriasis just *never* seems to get better." Again, the room of heads nodded in agreement. "I think I know why it is not getting better," he explained. The entire audience grew silent, listening with anticipation, their heads peered forward and eyes wide open, eager to hear why scalp psoriasis is so difficult to treat. "Because you are not putting the medication on your head."

Across the entire room, everyone's heads dropped to their chests as they let out a sigh of catharsis. "Yes," they thought, "I have not been using the medication, and it feels so good to get it off my chest. I have been lying to my doctor about this for so long. It feels good to finally admit to a doctor that I have not really been using the medication."

26.1 Misconceptions about Scalp Psoriasis

Other explanations have been proposed for why scalp psoriasis is often refractory to treatment. One concept is that patients often scratch their scalp, inducing

Koebnerization of their psoriasis. Yet patients scratch other areas of their body, and this scratching does not produce psoriatic plaques in these areas that are as treatment resistant as scalp psoriasis. Another theory is that the scale of scalp psoriasis inhibits the penetration of topical agents. We should know this is not true. The normal scalp exhibits percutaneous absorption similar to the axilla (Maibach, 1973), and diseased skin has poor barrier function. Indeed, clinical trials have demonstrated that rapid relief of scalp psoriasis can be achieved with topical clobetasol without a concomitant keratolytic agent (Jarratt, 2004; Stein, 2005). Scalp psoriasis is one of the forms of psoriasis most sensitive to topical steroids; scalp psoriasis seems resistant to treatment because patients are "resistant" to applying the medication to their hair-bearing scalp.

26.2 A Thought Experiment

Scalp psoriasis is the mother of all poor adherence problems. Consider what it would take to apply a peanut oil product to your scalp. Imagine yourself in the bathroom trying to use the medication. It takes a considerable amount of time to spread it along your entire pre-moistened scalp, and it may involve some mess depending on where it drips. Imagine putting a shower cap on over the product. Now imagine placing your head on your pillow, sporting that shower cap, and experiencing the unpleasant sensation of your hair bathing in a greasy ointment, all while lying in bed next to your spouse, date, or some other person. Our lives are so busy already. How many of us would adhere to such a time-consuming, messy, and uncomfortable treatment? If a physician told us to follow this routine for a few months, how many of us would quickly give up, if we ever started at all?

26.3 Approaches to Improve Adherence in Scalp Psoriasis

26.3.1 Choosing the Correct Vehicle

We should begin with a single treatment; the more complex the regimen, the more difficult it will be for our patients to adhere to the treatment plan. Something fast acting, like a clobetasol product, would be a good choice. We should select an appropriate vehicle; there are many options—a solution, foam, shampoo, or oil, among others—but we should prescribe the one the patient prefers. In most situations, we prescribe generic clobetasol solution. For African American patients who find an alcohol-based solution drying or who are already using oil products on their scalp, a scalp oil steroid formulation may be best. For some patients, a shampoo-based clobetasol product may be preferred. Since most patients use shampoo anyway, recommending a clobetasol shampoo may add little, if any, burden to their daily routine (although it is recommended that the clobetasol shampoo be applied to a dry scalp and left in place for 15 minutes or so before rinsing out). It may be hard to believe that a short-contact agent such as a shampoo would suffice for scalp psoriasis, given how treatment-resistant scalp psoriasis can be. Nevertheless, clinical studies prove this approach is effective, and many patients find it convenient to use (Jarratt, 2004).

26.3.2 Shortening the Treatment Time Horizon

Because it is so tedious to apply topical agents to hair-bearing scalp, we should reduce the burden of treatment by limiting the treatment time horizon. We might encourage patients to use the medication twice a day for a mere three days. In a recent study, seven patients applied clobetasol lotion to their scalp twice daily for seven days and were told to expect phone calls three days after beginning treatment to follow up on the treatment progress (Rajabi-Estarabadi and Hasanzadeh, 2018); six of seven patients were satisfied with the results. Scalp psoriasis clears very quickly with clobetasol, as we learned from Skin Cap: " 'It's a miracle.' . . . Her psoriasis of the scalp, which had been modestly improved under our treatment for several months, was now gone. It had taken just four days" (Shelley and Shelley, 1997).

Speaking in the most caring and empathetic voice possible and with a caring hand on their shoulder, we might express to our patients, "We know it is going to be difficult. We know it is going to be time consuming. We need you to apply the medication twice a day. But it is only for three days. Come back to the office in three days, and we will see how you are doing. Now it may sting; in my experience, the stinging is a sign that it is working." If the patient lives far away or is too busy to return, we can provide them with our phone number, again expressing our concern for them, conveying our desire to help them avoid paying another co-pay, and asking them to call in three days to report their progress. Implementing some kind of contact after a short initial duration of treatment encourages patients to use the medication well, gets them in the habit of using the medication, and lets them see how fast the medication can work. Giving them our phone number engenders trust that further facilitates adherence. It would be much as if the dentist told them, "I am really worried about your gums. Floss your teeth twice a day, and I will see you back here in the office in three days." Patients would floss more during those three days than they might normally do in an entire month!

26.3.3 Simplifying the Treatment Regimen

One patient visited the office reporting that her scalp psoriasis had become resistant to three forms of clobetasol therapy—solution, foam, and shampoo—simultaneously. Rather than adding yet another medication, we recommended that she focus solely on using the shampoo. We instructed her to apply it twice a day for three days and then call us to report her results. A bit peeved, she asked, "Do you not understand? I am already using that medication, and it does not work." We expressed our understanding and explained that the other two agents might have been working "at cross purposes" with the shampoo. We then asked her to trust us and advised her again simply to use the shampoo for three days. She called back in three days, overjoyed that the scalp lesions had essentially vanished. Had the other two medications been working at cross purposes with the shampoo? They were, in a sense, because the complexity of her original regimen made adherence nearly impossible.

26.3.4 Recruiting a Friend or Partner

Scalp psoriasis is very difficult for our patients to treat by themselves. Women's hair may have as much as 60 times more surface area than their scalp, so most of the topical agent likely ends up on their hair unless they are extremely careful. We had one teenage patient with a very full head of hair who visited us for treatment-resistant scalp psoriasis accompanied by her mother; the referring dermatologist wanted to know if the patient needed biologic treatment (etanercept) for the scalp psoriasis. We recommended topical clobetasol and a follow-up call in three days. After three days, we spoke with the patient's mother who said that the scalp was just a little bit better. We said the improvement was encouraging, and they should continue the treatment for another three days. We spoke again then, and the mother reported the scalp was no better. We asked who was applying the medication, and the mother reported that her teenage daughter was doing it herself. We asked Mom to apply the medication to the daughter's scalp for the next three days. When we spoke after those three days, the mother reported the scalp was now clear. She also told us that we need to let people know that treating scalp psoriasis is a two-person job.

In many ways, applying topical therapy for scalp psoriasis is akin to getting our hair colored. The hair is separated down to the scalp, and one row of medication is applied. Hair is successively shifted over, exposing another row of scalp, and the medication is applied again. Following this process for the entire scalp requires two individuals. We might tell our patients, "You have so much hair that you could not possibly apply the medication on your own, so have someone else help you." Patients love to be told they have a lot of hair, and this compliment strengthens the patient–physician relationship. Furthermore, involving two people—one with the disease and another who applies the medication—doubles the odds that at least one of them exhibits the obsessive-compulsive traits that facilitate effective use of the medication.

26.4 Concluding Thoughts

Witnessing a patient with treatment-resistant scalp psoriasis rapidly improve is one of the most gratifying aspects of dermatology. Once we understand that scalp psoriasis is refractory because of poor adherence, we can help our patients' lesions improve quickly and easily.

Section 7

Final Thoughts

DOI: 10.1201/9781003367628-33

27

Poor Adherence Is Not All Bad

Poor adherence is ubiquitous in dermatology and remains a common cause of treatment failure and frustration among both physicians and patients. Nevertheless, poor adherence is not all bad. One of the best aspects of poor adherence is that it limits the adverse effects of treatment.

Potent topical corticosteroids such as clobetasol and betamethasone are commonly prescribed in dermatology and can induce cutaneous atrophy. It is a wonder that adverse effects occur so rarely—or perhaps it should not be a wonder. The main reason we do not see these adverse effects very frequently is likely poor adherence.

It is difficult enough to get patients to take pills for a week. Getting patients to apply topical agents for the long-term management of chronic skin disease represents an even more daunting challenge. Even when their skin disease is intensely bothersome, they may not use their medication. The vast majority of patients stop using their medication as their disease improves. In this sense, poor adherence represents a natural technique for limiting the adverse effects of topical agents.

There are exceptions, though, such as obsessive-compulsive patients who might continue using topical medications even after they are no longer needed. Atrophy commonly occurs in areas with thin, delicate skin, such as the face, axilla, or groin. However, atrophy can also occur in areas where patients are obsessed about their disease—for example, the shins in women—to the extent that they continue applying topical steroids after the lesions have already flattened. Indeed, if the induration and scale have disappeared but the patient continues to use topical steroids for residual macular erythema, atrophy may occur. This outcome is certainly unusual, and such a finding would be incredibly rare in scalp psoriasis.

DOI: 10.1201/9781003367628-34

28

Conclusions

Being cynical about patients' adherence is likely a good thing that will help us give our patients better care, reduce their suffering, and improve their outcomes. We might consider changing what we call "self-administered" medications to "self-non-administered" medications. We should not speak of patients taking their medication unless we watched them do it. It would be more appropriate to say, "The patient says they are taking the medication"; "The patient was prescribed these medications"; "The patient claims to be taking these medications"; or, our favorite, particularly when the medication is not working as we expect it should, "Allegedly, the patient is taking drugs X, Y, and Z." Saying "The patient is on drugs X, Y, and Z" may mislead us into thinking they are taking the treatments as prescribed.

The costs of poor adherence and patient-proclaimed treatment failures are significant. Frequent clinic visits and half-full bottles of medications add to the direct costs of chronic skin diseases such as atopic dermatitis and psoriasis. The continued suffering of the patient is an even bigger cost.

Who is at fault for poor adherence? We are. We have so many tools at our disposal to get patients to use their medications, but we often fail to apply them. At the foundation, we should establish a physician–patient relationship that engenders trust, and we should incorporate some form of accountability into the treatment plan. Our treatment approaches should be simple and tailored to the preferences of each patient. On top of that, we can use a variety of powerful yet simple psychological tools to further encourage good adherence.

Medicine in general (and dermatology in particular) is an interesting field on many levels. For those new to the field, the number of diseases is formidable. The wide array of treatments we use adds another layer of complexity to the management of skin diseases. Yet within a few years, we become adept at making the right diagnosis and choosing the appropriate treatment within milliseconds of seeing the rash. Clinical practice remains interesting, though, because our patients provide a bottomless wealth of novelty and challenges.

The obstacles associated with patient adherence make dermatology a more challenging field. The complexity of doing what we must do to get patients to use their medications raises the challenge and joy of successful dermatology practice. There is no single approach that will work for all of us. Patient adherence is very complex and is influenced by a myriad of factors. Figuring out how to get our patients to use the medications we prescribe is partly art, partly science, and all fun.

Nevertheless, we can make certain generalizations. First, we ought to assume that patients will likely have trouble using their medications regularly. For this reason, we must ensure that patients recognize that we are trustworthy, caring physicians

DOI: 10.1201/9781003367628-35

committed to helping them get well. We should also establish accountability, especially early in the treatment period when patients are developing the habit of taking the medication. We should involve patients in the choice of treatment, proposing treatment regimens and delivery systems with which they are comfortable. We should avoid overstating the risks of adverse events and instead use the risks to our advantage when appropriate by letting patients know that they are a sign the drug is working. We should also formulate treatment plans conducive to rapid improvement. Once patients see that the medication works, they will be more likely to continue using it, at least as needed. Otherwise, the patient will observe limited initial improvement and will be more likely to give up on the medication altogether.

New drug development offers great promise for our field. But we already have medications in our armamentarium that can benefit the overwhelming majority of our patients. Helping them use the agents we can prescribe now may be far more effective (and less costly) than developing the next innovative therapy, particularly if they don't adhere to the new one any better than they did the old one. Whether we are the first dermatologist to see the patient or the sixth, we must remember that our responsibilities include more than simply making the right diagnosis and prescribing the right therapy. We must also do our best to get patients to use their medications.

References

Ali SM, Brodell RT, Balkrishnan R, Feldman SR. Poor adherence to treatments: a fundamental principle of dermatology. *Arch Dermatol.* 2007 Jul;143(7):912–15.

Alinia H, Feldman SR. Assessing medication adherence using indirect self-report. *JAMA Dermatol.* 2014;150(8):813–4.

Alinia H, Moradi Tuchayi S, Smith JA, Richardson IM, Bahrami N, Jaros SC, Sandoval LF, Farhangian ME, Anderson KL, Huang KE, Feldman SR. Long-term adherence to topical psoriasis treatment can be abysmal: a 1-year randomized intervention study using objective electronic adherence monitoring. *Br J Dermatol.* 2017 Mar;176(3):759–64.

Anderson KL, Dothard EH, Huang KE, Feldman SR. Frequency of primary nonadherence to acne treatment. *JAMA Dermatol.* 2015 Jun;151(6):623–6.

Baldwin HE. Tricks for improving compliance with acne treatment. *Dermatol Ther.* 2006 Jul–Aug;19(4):224–36.

Balkrishnan R. The importance of medication adherence in improving chronic-disease related outcomes: what we know and what we need to further know. *Med Care.* 2005 Jun;43(6):517–20.

Balkrishnan R, Carroll CL, Camacho FT, Feldman SR. Electronic monitoring of medication adherence in skin disease: results of a pilot study. *J Am Acad Dermatol.* 2003 Oct;49(4):651–4.

Barankin B. *Dermographies: Autobiographies in Dermatology, Volume 2.* Nova Scotia, Canada: Community Books, 2006.

Barfod TS, Hecht FM, Rubow C, Gerstoft J. Physicians' communication with patients about adherence to HIV medication in San Francisco and Copenhagen: a qualitative study using grounded theory. *BMC Health Serv Res.* 2006;6:154.

Bashyam AM, Cuellar-Barboza A, Ghamrawi RI, Feldman SR. Placebo tailoring improves patient satisfaction of treatment plans in atopic dermatitis. *J Am Acad Dermatol.* 2020 Sep;83(3):944–6.

Bashyam AM, Cuellar-Barboza A, Masicampo EJ, Feldman SR. Framing atopic dermatitis topical medication application site discomfort as a signal of efficacy improves willingness to continue use. *J Am Acad Dermatol.* 2020 Dec;83(6):1773–5.

Beutner K, Chakrabarty A, Lemke S, Yu K. An intra-individual randomized safety and efficacy comparison of clobetasol propionate 0.05% spray and its vehicle in the treatment of plaque psoriasis. *J Drugs Dermatol.* 2006 Apr;5(4):357–60.

Bhatia S, Landier W, Hageman L, Kim H, Chen Y, Crews KR, Evans WE, Bostrom B, Casillas J, Dickens DS, Maloney KW, Neglia JP, Ravindranath Y, Ritchey AK, Wong FL, Relling MV. 6MP adherence in a multiracial cohort of children with acute lymphoblastic leukemia: a children's oncology group study. *Blood.* 2014 Oct 9;124(15):2345–53.

Brown KK, Rehmus WE, Kimball AB. Determining the relative importance of patient motivations for nonadherence to topical corticosteroid therapy in psoriasis. *J Am Acad Dermatol.* 2006 Oct;55(4):607–13.

Burns T, Breathnach S, Cox N, Griffiths C. *Rook's Textbook of Dermatology*, 8th Ed. Hoboken, NJ: Wiley-Blackwell, 2010.

Carroll CL, Clarke J, Camacho F, Balkrishnan R, Feldman SR. Topical tacrolimus ointment combined with 6% salicylic acid gel for plaque psoriasis treatment. *Arch Dermatol*. 2005 Jan;141(1):43–6.

Carroll CL, Feldman SR, Camacho FT, Manuel JC, Balkrishnan R. Adherence to topical therapy decreases during the course of an 8-week psoriasis clinical trial: commonly used methods of measuring adherence to topical therapy overestimate actual use. *J Am Acad Dermatol*. 2004 Aug;51(2):212–16.

Davis SA, Feldman SR. Using Hawthorne effects to improve adherence in clinical practice: lessons from clinical trials. *JAMA Dermatol*. 2013 Apr;149(4):490–1.

Davis SA, Feldman SR. *An Illustrated Dictionary of Behavioral Economics for Healthcare Professionals*. North Charleston, SC: CreateSpace, 2014.

Devine F, Edwards T, Feldman SR. Barriers to treatment: describing them from a different perspective. *Patient Prefer Adherence*. 2018 Jan 17;12:129–33.

Feldman SR. Effectiveness of clobetasol propionate spray 0.05% added to other stable treatments: add-on therapy in the COBRA trial. *Cutis*. 2007 Nov;80(5 Suppl):20–8.

Feldman SR. Context and contrast. *J Dermatolog Treat*. 2008;19(4):197–8.

Feldman SR. Advances in and hope for the treatment of parasitosis. *J Dermatolog Treat*. 2016;27(3):197.

Feldman SR, Brown KL, Heald P. 'Coral reef' psoriasis: a marker of resistance to topical treatment. *J Dermatolog Treat*. 2008;19(5):257–8.

Feldman SR, Camacho FT, Krejci-Manwaring J, Carroll CL, Balkrishnan R. Adherence to topical therapy increases around the time of office visits. *J Am Acad Dermatol*. 2007 Jul;57(1):81–3.

Feldman SR, Chen GJ, Hu JY, Fleischer AB. Effects of systematic asymmetric discounting on physician-patient interactions: a theoretical framework to explain poor compliance with lifestyle counseling. *BMC Med Inform Decis Mak*. 2002 Nov 25;2:8.

Feldman SR, Dempsey JR, Grummer S, Chen JG, Fleischer AB. Implications of a utility model for ultraviolet exposure behavior. *J Am Acad Dermatol*. 2001 Nov;45(5):718–22.

Fenerty SD, O'Neill JL, Gustafson CJ, Feldman SR. Maternal adherence factors in the treatment of pediatric atopic dermatitis. *JAMA Dermatol*. 2013;149(2):229–31.

Fleischer AB Jr. Black box warning for topical calcineurin inhibitors and the death of common sense. *Dermatol Online J*. 2006 Oct 31;12(6):2.

Franz TJ, Lehman PA, Feldman SR, Spellman MC. Bioavailability of clobetasol propionate in different vehicles. *Skin Pharmacol Appl Skin Physiol*. 2003 Jul–Aug;16(4):212–16.

Habif TP. *Clinical Dermatology: A Color Guide to Diagnosis and Therapy*, 5th Ed. Maryland Heights, MO: Mosby, 2009.

Housman TS, Keil KA, Mellen BG, McCarty MA, Fleischer AB Jr, Feldman SR. The use of 0.25% zinc pyrithione spray does not enhance the efficacy of clobetasol propionate 0.05% foam in the treatment of psoriasis. *J Am Acad Dermatol*. 2003 Jul;49(1):79–82.

Housman TS, Mellen BG, Rapp SR, Fleischer AB Jr, Feldman SR. Patients with psoriasis prefer solution and foam vehicles: a quantitative assessment of vehicle preference. *Cutis*. 2002 Dec;70(6):327–32.

Jarratt M, Breneman D, Gottlieb AB, Poulin Y, Liu Y, Foley V. Clobetasol propionate shampoo 0.05%: a new option to treat patients with moderate to severe scalp psoriasis. *J Drugs Dermatol.* 2004 Jul–Aug;3(4):367–73.

Johnson MC, Oussedik E, Huang WW, Kammrath LK, Feldman SR. Anecdote increases patient willingness to take a biologic medication for psoriasis. *Cutis.* 2021 Aug;108(2S):20–4.

Kahn JM, Stevenson K, Beauchemin M, Koch VB, Cole PD, Welch JJG, Gage-Bouchard E, Karsenty C, Silverman LB, Kelly KM, Bona K. Oral Mercaptopurine adherence in pediatric acute lymphoblastic leukemia: a survey study from the Dana-Farber cancer institute acute lymphoblastic leukemia consortium. *J Pediatr Hematol Oncol Nurs.* 2022 Jan–Feb;40(1):17–23.

Kaminska E, Patel I, Dabade TS, Chang J, Qureshi AA, O'Neill JL, Balkrishnan R, Feldman SR. Comparing the lifetime risks of TNF-alpha inhibitor use to common benchmarks of risk. *J Dermatolog Treat.* 2013 Apr;24(2):101–6.

Krejci-Manwaring J, Johnson KP, McCarty MA, Carroll CL, Hartle J, Manuel J, Balkrishnan R, Fleischer A Jr, Feldman SR. Comparison of different compliance behaviors in a clinical trial. *Cutis.* 2007 May;79(5):379–81.

Krejci-Manwaring J, McCarty MA, Camacho F, Carroll CL, Johnson K, Manuel J, Balkrishnan R, Hartle J, Fleischer A Jr, Feldman SR. Adherence with topical treatment is poor compared with adherence with oral agents: implications for effective clinical use of topical agents. *J Am Acad Dermatol.* 2006 May;54(5 Suppl):S235–6.

Krejci-Manwaring J, Tusa MG, Carroll C, Camacho F, Kaur M, Carr D, Fleischer AB Jr, Balkrishnan R, Feldman SR. Stealth monitoring of adherence to topical medication: adherence is very poor in children with atopic dermatitis. *J Am Acad Dermatol.* 2007 Feb;56(2):211–16.

Landier W, Chen Y, Hageman L, Kim H, Bostrom BC, Casillas JN, Dickens DS, Evans WE, Maloney KW, Mascarenhas L, Ritchey AK, Termuhlen AM, Carroll WL, Relling MV, Wong FL, Bhatia S. Comparison of self-report and electronic monitoring of 6MP intake in childhood ALL: a children's oncology group study. *Blood.* 2017 Apr 6;129(14):1919–26.

Lebwohl M, Colon LE. The evolving role of topical treatments in adjunctive therapy for moderate to severe plaque psoriasis. *Cutis.* 2007 Nov;80(5 Suppl):29–40.

Lewis DJ, Cardwell LA, Feldman SR. Applying behavioural economics to psoriasis treatment: interventions to improve patient adherence to biologics. *J Eur Acad Dermatol Venereol.* 2018 Feb;32(2):e65–6.

Lewis DJ, Feldman SR. Rapid, successful treatment of atopic dermatitis recalcitrant to topical corticosteroids. *Pediatr Dermatol.* 2018 Mar;35(2):278–9.

Luersen K, Davis SA, Kaplan SG, Abel TD, Winchester WW, Feldman SR. Sticker charts: a method for improving adherence to treatment of chronic diseases in children. *Pediatr Dermatol.* 2012 Jul–Aug;29(4):403–8.

Maibach HI, Stoughton RB. Topical corticosteroids. *Med Clin North Am.* 1973 Sep;57(5):1253–64.

Marks VJ, Hutchison R, Todd M. Service excellence in dermatology. *Semin Cutan Med Surg.* 2004 Sep;23(3):207–12.

Nelms H. *Magic and Showmanship: A Handbook for Conjurers.* Mineola, NY: Dover Publications Inc., 1969.

Okwundu N, Cardwell L, Cline A, Richardson I, Feldman SR. Is topical treatment effective for psoriasis in patients who failed topical treatment? *J Dermatolog Treat.* 2021 Feb;32(1):41–4.

Okwundu N, Cardwell LA, Cline A, Unrue EL, Richardson IM, Feldman SR. Topical corticosteroids for treatment-resistant atopic dermatitis. *Cutis.* 2018 Sep;102(3):205–9.

Oussedik E, Cardwell LA, Patel NU, Onikoyi O, Feldman SR. An anchoring-based intervention to increase patient willingness to use injectable medication in psoriasis. *JAMA Dermatol.* 2017 Sep;153(9):932–4.

Rajabi-Estarabadi A, Hasanzadeh H, Taheri A, Feldman SR, Firooz A. The efficacy of short-term clobetasol lotion in the treatment of scalp psoriasis. *J Dermatolog Treat.* 2018 Mar;29(2):111–15.

Rajpara AN, Landis ET, Feldman SR. Office evaluation: gaining a fresh perspective. *Dermatol.* 2012 May;20(5).

Reid DC, Kimball AB. Clobetasol propionate foam in the treatment of psoriasis. *Expert Opin Pharmacother.* 2005 Aug;6(10):1735–40.

Richards HL, Fortune DG, O'Sullivan TM, Main CJ, Griffiths CE. Patients with psoriasis and their compliance with medication. *J Am Acad Dermatol.* 1999 Oct;41(4):581–3.

Rohan JM, Drotar D, Alderfer M, Donewar CW, Ewing L, Katz ER, Muriel A. Electronic monitoring of medication adherence in early maintenance phase treatment for pediatric leukemia and lymphoma: identifying patterns of nonadherence. *J Pediatr Psychol.* 2015 Jan–Feb;40(1):75–84.

Rowlands CG, Danby FW. Histopathology of psoriasis treated with zinc pyrithione. *Am J Dermatopathol.* 2000 Jun;22(3):272–6.

Rubin BK. What does it mean when a patient says, "my asthma medication is not working?" *Chest.* 2004 Sep;126(3):972–81.

Saleem MD, Negus D, Feldman SR. Topical 0.25% desoximetasone spray efficacy for moderate to severe plaque psoriasis: a randomized clinical trial. *J Dermatolog Treat.* 2018 Feb;29(1):32–5.

Sandoval LF, Huang KE, Feldman SR. Adherence to ustekinumab in psoriasis patients. *J Drugs Dermatol.* 2013 Oct;12(10):1090–2.

Shelley WB, Shelley D. A dermatologic diary. Portrait of a practice. *Cutis.* 1997 Apr;59(4):181–2.

Siegfried EC, Jaworski JC, Hebert AA. Topical calcineurin inhibitors and lymphoma risk: evidence update with implications for daily practice. *Am J Clin Dermatol.* 2013 Jun;14(3):163–78.

Smith K. Skin cap: what have we learned, and when did we learn it? *Dermatol Online J.* 1997 Dec;3(2):11c.

Stein L. Clinical studies of a new vehicle formulation for topical corticosteroids in the treatment of psoriasis. *J Am Acad Dermatol.* 2005 Jul;53(1 Suppl):S39–49.

Storm A, Andersen SE, Benfeldt E, Serup J. One in 3 prescriptions are never redeemed: primary nonadherence in an outpatient clinic. *J Am Acad Dermatol.* 2008 Jul;59(1):27–33.

Storm A, Benfeldt E, Andersen SE, Andersen J. Basic drug information given by physicians is deficient, and patients' knowledge low. *J Dermatolog Treat.* 2009;20(4):190–3.

Swanson DL, Pittelkow MR, Benson LM, Hawkridge AM, Muddiman DC. Déjà vu all over again: skin cap still contains a high-potency glucocorticosteroid. *Arch Dermatol.* 2005 Jun;141(6):801–3.

Uhas AA, Camacho FT, Feldman SR, Balkrishnan R. The relationship between physician friendliness and caring, and patient satisfaction: findings from an internet-based survey. *Patient.* 2008 Apr 1;1(2):91–6.

Warino L, Balkrishnan R, Feldman SR. Clobetasol propionate for psoriasis: are ointments really more potent? *J Drugs Dermatol.* 2006 Jun;5(6):527–32.

Yentzer BA, Ade RA, Fountain JM, Clark AR, Taylor SL, Fleischer AB Jr, Feldman SR. Simplifying regimens promotes greater adherence and outcomes with topical acne medications: a randomized controlled trial. *Cutis.* 2010 Aug;86(2):103–8.

Yentzer BA, Alikhan A, Teuschler H, Williams LL, Tusa M, Fleischer AB Jr, Kaur M, Balkrishnan R, Feldman SR. An exploratory study of adherence to topical benzoyl peroxide in patients with acne vulgaris. *J Am Acad Dermatol.* 2009 May;60(5):879–80.

Yentzer BA, Camacho FT, Young T, Fountain JM, Clark AR, Feldman SR. Good adherence and early efficacy using desonide hydrogel for atopic dermatitis: results from a program addressing patient compliance. *J Drugs Dermatol.* 2010 Apr;9(4):324–9.

Yentzer BA, Gosnell AL, Clark AR, Pearce DJ, Balkrishnan R, Camacho FT, Young TA, Fountain JM, Fleischer AB Jr, Colón LE, Johnson LA, Preston N, Feldman SR. A randomized controlled pilot study of strategies to increase adherence in teenagers with acne vulgaris. *J Am Acad Dermatol.* 2011 Apr;64(4):793–5.

Yentzer BA, Hick J, Williams L, Inabinet R, Wilson R, Camacho FT, Russell GB, Feldman SR. Adherence to a topical regimen of 5-fluorouracil, 0.5%, cream for the treatment of actinic keratoses. *Arch Dermatol.* 2009 Feb;145(2):203–5.

Yentzer BA, Wood AA, Sagransky MJ, O'Neill JL, Clark AR, Williams LL, Feldman SR. An internet-based survey and improvement of acne treatment outcomes. *Arch Dermatol.* 2011 Oct;147(10):1223–4.

Zaghloul SS, Goodfield MJ. Objective assessment of compliance with psoriasis treatment. *Arch Dermatol.* 2004 Apr;140(4):408–14.

Index

Note: Page numbers in *italics* indicate a figure and page numbers in **bold** indicate a table on the corresponding page.